50 BEST SHORT HIKES
SAN DIEGO
2ND EDITION

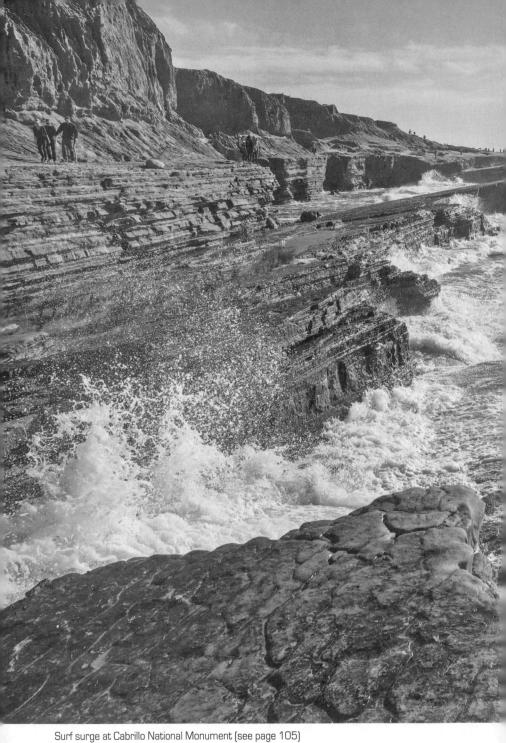

Surf surge at Cabrillo National Monument (see page 105)

50 BEST SHORT HIKES
SAN DIEGO
2ND EDITION

JERRY SCHAD
and
DON ENDICOTT

 WILDERNESS PRESS . . . *on the trail since 1967*

50 Best Short Hikes: San Diego
2nd EDITION 2018, 2nd printing 2022
Copyright © 2011 by Jerry Schad
Copyright © 2018 by Don Endicott
Interior and cover photos by Don Endicott, except where noted
Maps and cover design: Scott McGrew
Interior design: Annie Long

Library of Congress Cataloging-in-Publication Data

Names: Schad, Jerry, author. | Endicott, Don, author.
Title: 50 best short hikes : San Diego / [Jerry Schad, Don Endicott].
Other titles: Fifty best short hikes
Description: Second Edition. | Birmingham, Alabama : WILDERNESS PRESS
    . . . on the trail since 1967, [2018] | Includes index. | "Distributed by Publishers
    Group West"—T.p. verso.
Identifiers: LCCN 2017029448| ISBN 9780899978802 (paperback) | ISBN
    9780899978819 (ebook)
Subjects: LCSH: Hiking—California—San Diego—Guidebooks. | Backpacking—
    California—San Diego—Guidebooks. | Trails—California—San Diego—
    Guidebooks. | Outdoor recreation. | San Diego (Calif.)—Guidebooks.
Classification: LCC GV199.42.C22 S2668 2018 | DDC 796.5109794/985—dc23
LC record available at https://lccn.loc.gov/2017029448

Manufactured in the United States of America

Published by: **WILDERNESS PRESS**
    An imprint of AdventureKEEN
    2204 First Ave. S, Ste. 102
    Birmingham, AL 35233
    800-678-7006; FAX 877-374-9016

Visit wildernesspress.com for a complete listing of our books and for ordering information. Contact us at our website, at facebook.com/wildernesspress1967, or at twitter.com
/wilderness1967 with questions or comments. To find out more about who we are and
what we're doing, visit blog.wildernesspress.com.

Distributed by Publishers Group West

Front cover: Pools below Cabrillo Coastal Trail (see page 105)
Back cover: El Capitan viewed from east of Louis A. Stelzer County Park (see page 136)

Safety Notice
Though Wilderness Press and the authors have made every attempt to ensure that the
information in this book is accurate at press time, they are not responsible for any loss,
damage, injury, or inconvenience that may occur to anyone while using this book. You
are responsible for your own safety and health. The fact that a trail is described in this
book does not mean that it will be safe for you. Be aware that trail conditions can change
from day to day. Always check local conditions, know your own limitations, and consult
a map and compass.

To Jerry Schad, in appreciation of three decades of friendship and outdoor adventures, and my wife, Marilyn Endicott, my life partner, companion, and best friend.

50 Best Short Hikes: San Diego

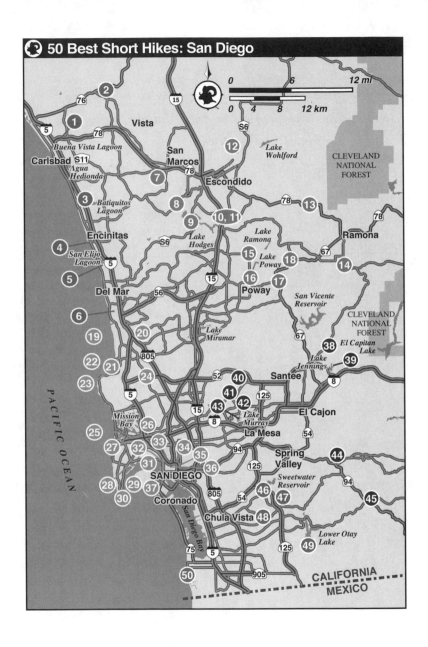

Contents

Acknowledgments

50 Best Short Hikes: San Diego contains a large amount of adapted and updated material from weekly or monthly columns researched and written by Jerry Schad that have appeared in various publications over the past 35 years. Versions of some of the material are included in the comprehensive guidebook *Afoot & Afield: San Diego County*, available in a fifth edition revised by Scott Turner. This new edition of *50 Best Short Hikes: San Diego* shares much of the same literary DNA with these other resources. I personally researched, rehiked, and recorded GPS tracks and waypoints for Jerry's original 50 best hikes to ensure accuracy and reflect changes in trail and habitat conditions since the first edition's original publication in 2011. Eventually, a total of 60 hikes were surveyed and 5 new hikes incorporated as replacements where construction projects or other impacts reduced the attractiveness of an original hike. My wife, Marilyn, joined me for a number of the shorter hikes and contributed support and encouragement throughout the endeavor. I thank Scott Turner for helping steer this opportunity my way and to Peg Reiter, Jerry's widow, for endorsing my coauthorship role. Scott graciously shared his experiences and tips associated with revising the fifth edition of *Afoot & Afield: San Diego County*, joined me for several of the hikes, and corresponded regularly as we traded notes on our two projects.

While it might seem unusual to acknowledge a coauthor, I am compelled to reflect on the many great—and characteristically physically challenging—times Jerry and I shared in the field going back to the early 1980s. Back then he was researching what eventually became San Diego's preeminent hiking guide, the first edition of *Afoot & Afield: San Diego County*. Jerry was ever fascinated with maps and all things relating to the natural world: plants, animals, and—perhaps his greatest passion—the night sky. He was deeply knowledgeable in these areas and erudite in sharing informed insights with others through written word, while leading day hikes or longer outings, and in the classroom. Jerry was a consummate photographer, and over the years we frequently shared memorable images with each other. Jerry was a friend to the end of his life. I will always remember and treasure our engaging conversations in his home throughout his last months after contracting irreversible cancer, reminiscing at times, but also sharing and discussing recent good reads, as well as his vision for this addition to his extensive publication portfolio. Jerry, thank you for leading the way toward a deeper appreciation of the very best outdoor San Diego has to offer. I hope you are pleased with this new edition of *50 Best Short Hikes: San Diego*.

Echoing Jerry's acknowledgments in the first edition, I am indebted to scores—too numerous to mention here—of friends, acquaintances, and rangers who have generously provided background information, past and present.

I would like to express my appreciation for several individuals at Wilderness Press: Tim Jackson was my primary contact, ably guiding this first-time author throughout the editorial and publication process. Prior to the first edition, Roslyn Bullas revived the 50 Best Short Hikes concept. Amber Kaye Henderson thoroughly and ably edited the text. Scott McGrew and Annie Long handled the book's cartography and design.

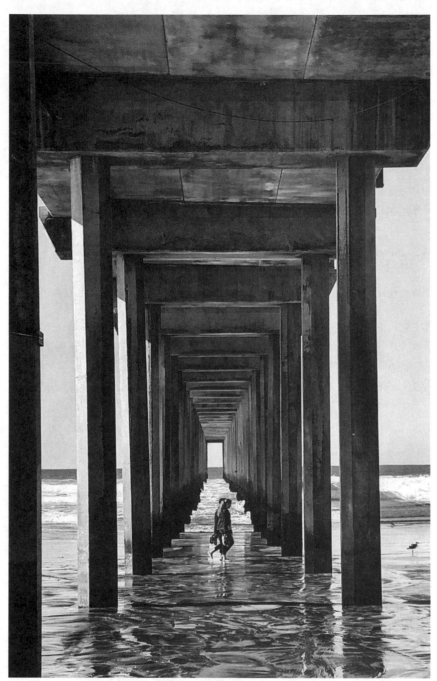
Looking out to sea beneath Scripps Pier (see page 78)

The Very Best Short Hikes

VERY BEST ARCHITECTURE AND HISTORY

33. Bankers Hill *San Diego's elite residents erected mansions in this exquisitely walkable neighborhood.*

36. Gaslamp Quarter *Stroll among San Diego's most complete collection of historic buildings, now part of the city's liveliest entertainment district.*

VERY BEST BIRD- AND WILDLIFE-WATCHING

5. San Elijo Lagoon *The waterway hosts birds of shoreline and coastal lagoon habitats, as well as small animals.*

43. Lake Murray *From hawks and ravens in the sky, to egrets and pelicans in the water, to coyotes and rabbits on the ground—Lake Murray has it all.*

50. Imperial Beach *At times, large flocks of seabirds congregate here.*

VERY BEST FOR DOG WALKING

8. Elfin Forest Recreational Reserve *Your pet (if physically fit) can roam in unlimited space.*

16. Lake Poway Loop *Both dogs and their masters/mistresses will enjoy this excellent exercise course.*

43. Lake Murray *The lake's wide shoreline path accommodates all users, including leashed pets.*

VERY BEST FOR EASY STROLLING

22. Coast Walk *Some unpaved trails, but mostly sidewalks, lead the way to La Jolla's best coastal vistas.*

29. Shelter Island *Feast your eyes on the San Diego Bay shoreline as you meander.*

34. Balboa Park's Central Mesa *The paved walk welcomes you into the park's most lavishly landscaped section.*

VERY BEST FOR RUNNING

4. Swami's Beach *Several sets of cliff-edge staircases draw runners for serious interval training.*

25. Circling Sail Bay *A near-flat breezy course parallels the shoreline of Mission Bay.*

32. The Embarcadero *A totally flat course features San Diego's best urban-coastal scenery.*

48. Rice Canyon *This mellow course winds down along an unspoiled coastal canyon.*

VERY BEST FOR SMALL CHILDREN

1. Hosp Grove *A sun-dappled eucalyptus forest is fun to explore.*

30. Cabrillo National Monument *The Whale Overlook and Old Point Loma Lighthouse, the tidepools at the south end of the Coastal Trail, and roaming interpretive rangers and volunteers delight young and not so young.*

37. Coronado Beach *From a small child's perspective, here is where an ocean of sand meets an ocean of seawater.*

VERY BEST SPRINGTIME WILDFLOWERS

19. Torrey Pines State Natural Reserve *Coastal-region wildflowers put on a flamboyant show.*

40. Oak Canyon *The wildflowers common to inland San Diego County are well represented here with an added bonus of two seasonal waterfalls.*

45. Hollenbeck Canyon *Wet winters yield early-spring wildflower spectacles.*

VERY BEST VISTAS

17. Iron Mountain *The summit vantage encompasses 360 degrees from ocean shore to mountain crest.*

19. Torrey Pines State Natural Reserve *The reserve offers the most beautiful melding of land and sea in San Diego County.*

23. Soledad Mountain *You'll find superlative urban and coastline vistas.*

30. Cabrillo National Monument *Walk the Coastal and Bayside Trails for spectacular ocean and San Diego Bay scenery, particularly in late afternoon.*

42. Cowles Mountain *It features the most comprehensive views of urban and suburban San Diego.*

44. McGinty Mountain *One of East County's signature high points, McGinty Mountain offers a 360-degree skyline panorama that a soaring hawk or eagle might see.*

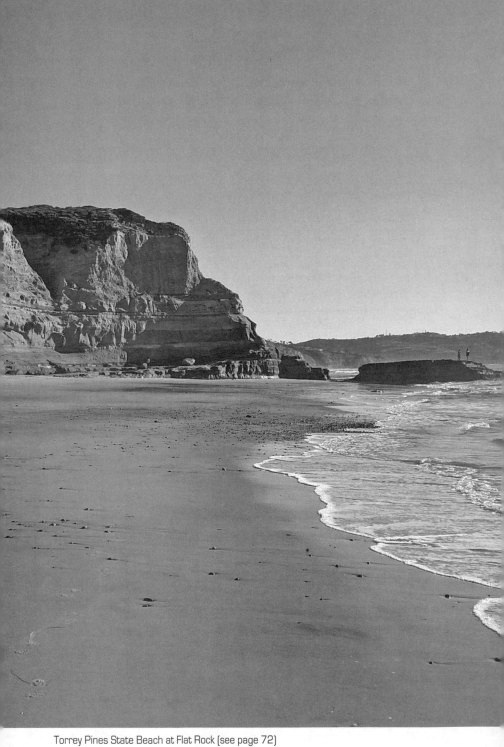

Torrey Pines State Beach at Flat Rock (see page 72)

INTRODUCTION

Sunshine. Water and waves. Blue skies and mild temperatures. Sports and leisure. This list of attributes pretty much sums up the image that San Diego projects to the world—and that image is true!

Tourists visiting San Diego for the first time are amazed at the sheer magnitude of park spaces and recreational venues. Everywhere, it seems, people are engaged in outdoor recreation. People are not only swimming, surfing, boating, fishing, picnicking, golfing, and playing tennis, but they're also running, biking, skating, and *walking*.

The focus of *50 Best Short Hikes: San Diego* is all about walking, and doing it on the most outstanding 50 trails in this metropolitan region. The selection is so varied that you can match the trail to your time, your mood, your energy level, and even to what shoes you're wearing—or not: the trail surfaces throughout San Diego range from concrete and asphalt to dirt footpaths and sandy beaches.

Geographically, the hike selections include the suburbs and nearby communities that surround the city of San Diego: just picture the Pacific Ocean coastline from Oceanside in the north to Imperial Beach near the Mexican border. Add to that the various bay and river shorelines. Then color in the hills, canyons, and valleys stretching east up to—within the parameters of this guidebook—about 20 miles inland from the coast. (San Diego County actually extends much farther east than that, encompassing mile-high-plus mountain ranges and a vast desert region. Those remote, eastern areas are covered in detail in a companion book published by Wilderness Press titled *Afoot & Afield: San Diego County*.)

The roughly 1,000 square miles of landscape covered in this book offer a year-round mild climate, easy to moderate types of terrain suitable for almost any hiker, and amazingly varied scenery. To put icing on the cake, you may reach the trailheads by car via one of the world's most efficient roadway systems. In the next few paragraphs, let's focus on these superlative claims.

Coastal San Diego County's weather is often tagged as Mediterranean: generally warm and sunny, and winter-wet, summer-dry. Despite San Diego's low latitude within the 48 contiguous states, a cool Pacific current moving south along California's coast helps keep the area pleasantly air-conditioned on summer days. Mountain ranges north and east hold cold-air masses at bay during the winter. The bottom line is that daytime coastal temperatures nearly always hover within the 60°F–75°F range. The winter-wet season isn't all that wet: only about 10 inches of rainfall per year, most coming in December–February, and there is no snow! Farther inland, up to 20 miles from the coast for these hiking routes, temperatures aren't quite as mild, with some summer days reaching the 90s, and some winter nights dipping below freezing.

However, where and when heat is a factor, this guidebook coaches you to hike in early mornings or late afternoons—or to save those areas for fall, winter, or spring excursions. And as it is all about day hikes in these pages, you won't have to concern yourself with bundling up in sleeping bags. (Well, a few trails in this book are suggested for enchanting full-moon excursions, but night hiking is recommended only in comfortable weather.)

Another comfort factor is elevation, which is the leading determinant for easy versus difficult trails. While coastal San Diego County isn't highly mountainous, the landscape does rise and fall in a dramatic fashion here and there. As a consequence, the most demanding trails in this book may involve hundreds (but never thousands) of feet of elevation gain and loss—cumulative elevation change—over the course of the hike.

Your payoff for elevation gain in this region is views, views, and views. San Diego is not only highly scenic, but it's also scenically diverse. One route offers a vista of waves and ocean bluffs, while a nearby trail darts into a fragrant eucalyptus grove, and yet another threads through oak woods next to a trickling stream. One trailside panorama encompasses square miles of boulder-frosted mountainsides, while an urban vista frames downtown San Diego's glimmering skyline over the sparkling waters of San Diego Bay.

For a healthy mix of flora and fauna, city and country, you're in the right place when you hike here. The whole of San Diego County (4,526 square miles) is home to more than 2,000 species of native plants and has more biodiversity than any area of comparable size within the continental United States. Some 500 species of birds have been spotted in San Diego County, more than most other counties or parishes in the nation, including Hawaii. Among the 50 routes covered in this book, you will come upon enough living things to not disappoint. And the hike descriptions tell you what to

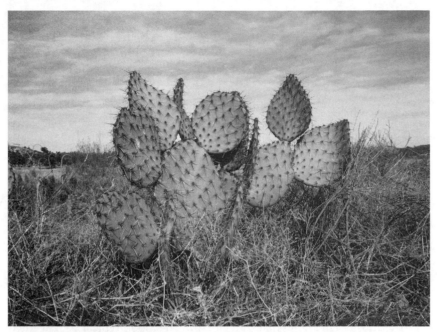

Coast prickly pear cactus

especially look for among plant and animal species along that trail. Also among these 50 routes, at least a quarter of the hikes weave through some of San Diego's most interesting urban neighborhoods. You'll enjoy the inner city's treasure trove of historical, architectural, and cultural points of interest.

Lastly, from and around the city core, San Diego's freeway system reaches out to nearly every suburb of consequence. That means that parks and open space areas on the suburban fringe are easily accessible. Barring traffic tie-ups on weekday mornings and afternoons, nearly every hike in this book is accessible within an hour or less of driving from the heart of the city.

USING THIS BOOK

The audience for this book is twofold: One is local residents who seek fresh walking routes—or who want to explore their own metro backyards more thoroughly. The other is tourists or business travelers who want a quick post-afternoon-meeting or post-sightseeing bit of exercise.

Whatever made *you* reach for this book, *50 Best Short Hikes: San Diego* will entice you to the area's best trails and pathways that are no more than 8 miles in distance and that have no severe elevation gains. Most of the hikes actually fall within the 1- to 4-mile range, which makes them quite suitable for casual hikers.

The most challenging hikes included in this book typically are located inland, rather far from the most densely settled and tourist-friendly sections of San Diego. Such routes may be perfect for half-daylong jaunts, especially on weekends. In some cases, you may have physical limitations to consider. In others, perhaps small children will accompany your walk. Whatever your particular needs or interests, there are hikes for you. Peruse "The Very Best Short Hikes" section on page xii to help you decide where to start.

To select hikes geographically, check the locator map on page vi. It depicts all five regions that are covered in this book and pinpoints the location of each of the 50 numbered hikes. The regional designations—Coastal North County, Inland North County, Coastal & Central San Diego, East County, and South County—are fairly common terms around San Diego. They refer to the metropolitan area of greater San Diego, not to the whole of San Diego County. (The latter includes about 2 million acres of remote mountains and desert that make up the true eastern half of the county, as well as Camp Pendleton, a large Marine Corps base on the county's northernmost coast.) In addition to their positions on the overall locator map, the five regions cited earlier each have a map and brief introduction preceding the trail profiles for that area. See page 9 for the map legend.

To select hikes based on elevation, please note that the "Elevation Range" in each hike profile's at-a-glance information refers to the highest and lowest elevation reached on that hike. For hikes involving a substantial amount of *cumulative* elevation gain and loss during the trip—meaning that you'll walk up and down a lot—such ascents and descents are noted in the main hike description.

STAYING SAFE

Every route in this book is safe in the sense that it is a designated public trail or access route, and it is typically popular with other users. Still, you must always be mindful of trail conditions that can change over time and due to weather.

Trails profiled herein vary from dead flat and paved to steep, rutty, and rocky. Please carefully read each trail description before you set out on any of these 50 hikes, and prepare for all of those on uneven surfaces by wearing hiking boots or sturdy walking shoes. If you know that you do not have a good sense of balance, please avoid hikes that could put you at risk of falling.

An example for such caution is the popular route up Cowles Mountain (Hike 42, page 150), the highest point in the city of San Diego. Though there are well over 100,000 separate ascents yearly up the 1.4-mile main trail, the billions of past footsteps on the unpaved path have worn deep

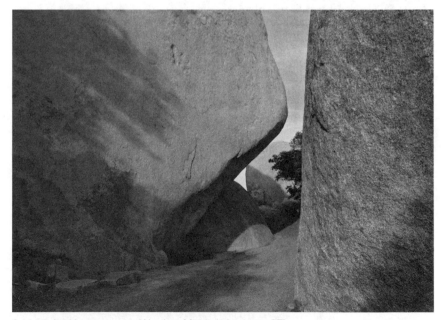

A narrow boulder passage on Woodson Mountain (see page 67)

grooves into the bedrock of the mountainside, creating an obstacle course of jutting rocks. The danger of tripping and falling isn't such a factor on the ascent, but it is more so on the descent, where stepping down on an uneven surface can result in a fall or a twisted ankle.

In general, you should be as mindful of precautions for these hikes as you are for any trail trekking:

- For all but the very short hikes, wear a lightweight backpack for carrying plenty of water and some snacks. Lack of adequate drinking water can sometimes be a critical issue on any of the hikes located in the hotter, inland areas. It's best to avoid inland hikes anytime the sun is high in the sky during the warmer months of the year. Walking will not be enjoyable at those times anyway.

- Your backpack is a good receptacle for extra clothing as well. Because inland San Diego County experiences wider swings in day and night temperatures than coastal areas, layering your attire is a good idea: take along two or more middleweight outer garments rather than relying on a single heavy or bulky jacket to keep you comfortable at all times.

- Raingear, however, finds only occasional use on the coastal trails of San Diego. Usually, there's plenty of advance warning when a rainstorm is brewing; it is highly unusual for fair weather to turn stormy within a short period of time. But always check the weather forecast.

- When the sun is shining (which is most of the time in this region), use sunglasses, wear long-sleeve tops, and apply sunscreen to your exposed skin. The higher the sun is in the sky, the more intense the solar ultraviolet. A broad-brimmed hat is highly recommended, with any head protection (for example, a ball cap or head scarf) better than none. Also, the greater the sun exposure, the greater the danger of dehydration, so fill up those water bottles and drink frequently!

- Don't forget to charge up and carry a cell phone before you set out on the walk. Still, do not forget that there are occasional dead zones for cell phone signals once you get away from populated places or well-traveled highways. Thus, as with all hiking, it is wise to let someone know where you are headed and when you expect to return.

- Hikers on the more remote trails in this book might want to store a flashlight in their backpacks (if there's any chance of being caught on the trail after dark); a map; a GPS unit or cell phone map application (for fun, as well as for navigation); a whistle (for signaling); and a first aid kit.

- Here and there, especially on trails following the small streams and through oak woodlands, poison oak growth can be copious.

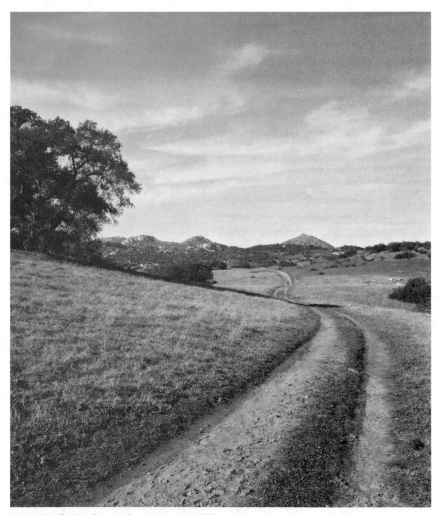

Valley View Trail at Barnett Ranch (see page 55)

Learn to recognize poison oak's distinctive three-leafed structure, and avoid touching it with skin or clothing. Poison oak loses its leaves during the winter (usually December–March in San Diego), but don't let that catch you unawares. The plant still retains some of the toxic oil in its stems, and it can be extra hazardous in winter because it is harder to identify and avoid.

◘ Rattlesnakes occasionally appear along the nonurban trails featured in this book. Typically, these creatures are as interested in avoiding contact with you as you are with them. But watch carefully where you put your feet, and especially your hands, during the warmer months, as you never want to startle a rattler. Most encounters between rattlesnakes and hikers occur in April and May, when snakes are out and about after a long hibernation period.

◘ Ticks also are an occasional problem, primarily on—again—the nonurban trails. They cling to the branches of shrubbery and wait for any warm-blooded host to wander by. If you can't avoid brushing against vegetation along the trail, be sure to check yourself for ticks frequently. Upon finding a host, a tick will usually crawl upward in search of a protected spot, where it will try to attach itself. If you can be aware of the slightest irritation on your body, you'll usually intercept ticks long before they attempt to latch on. Consider wearing light-colored long pants if you expect to encounter ticks, as it is easier to spot them quickly and flick them off before they find your skin.

◘ Mountain lion encounters are possible in the San Diego region, but this situation is extremely rare anywhere in San Diego County and especially along the inland-area trails covered in this book. Do, however, keep in mind that you should never run from any predatory animal. Make yourself look large. Gather together any children who are hiking with you. Do not act fearful. Pick up and throw rocks in the unlikely event that a lion doesn't immediately dash off, as they usually do (not only are mountain lion encounters rare, they typically last only a few seconds). Do anything to convince the animal that you are not its prey.

LEAVE NO TRACE

This guidebook's focus on short hikes within the radius of a major US city does not disregard the importance of preserving the natural environment.

Whether you're walking less than a mile through a city park or on an 8-mile backcountry route, please don't overlook your responsibility for your surroundings. Aside from common-sense prohibitions that anyone reading this book likely upholds against littering and vandalism, here are a few pointers:

▣ Never take shortcuts across trail switchbacks. This practice may save you some traveling distance, but it breaks down the trail tread and hastens erosion.

▣ Collecting minerals, plants, animals, and historic or prehistoric artifacts without a special permit is generally prohibited in most jurisdictions. That means common things too, such as pinecones, wildflowers, and lizards. These should be left for all visitors to enjoy—and for the lizards to continue enjoying in their own habitats.

▣ Take note of the signs and information kiosks at the beginning of each walk or hike, and heed all rules and precautions.

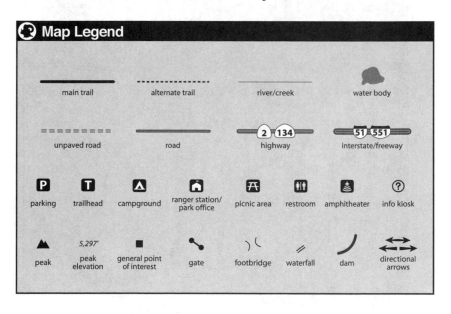

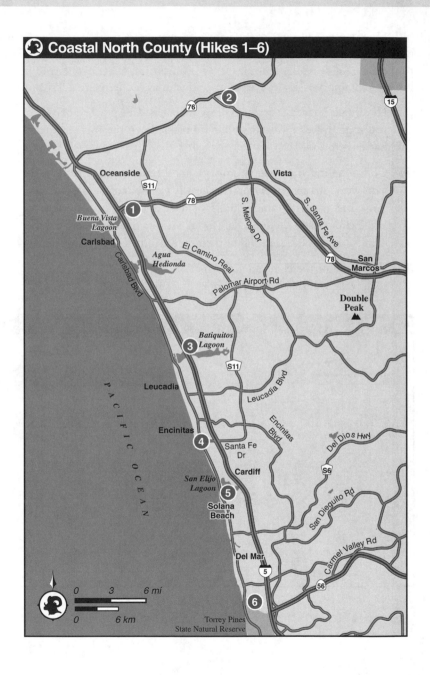

Coastal North County (Hikes 1–6)

76 ②

15

Oceanside

Vista

S11

78

S. Melrose Dr

S. Santa Fe Ave

①

Buena Vista Lagoon

Carlsbad

Carlsbad Blvd

Agua Hedionda

El Camino Real

78

San Marcos

Palomar Airport Rd

Double Peak

Batiquitos Lagoon ③

S11

Leucadia Blvd

P A C I F I C

Leucadia

Encinitas Blvd

Encinitas

④ Santa Fe Dr

Del Dios Hwy

San Elijo Lagoon ⑤

Cardiff

S6

O C E A N

Solana Beach

San Dieguito Rd

Del Mar

5

Carmel Valley Rd

56

0   3   6 mi

0   6 km

⑥

Torrey Pines State Natural Reserve

COASTAL NORTH COUNTY

Coastal North County's signature feature is a 20-mile-long, nearly unbroken strand of beaches and shoreline communities. From north to south, they are Oceanside, Carlsbad, Leucadia, Encinitas, Cardiff, Solana Beach, and Del Mar. Compared to the more densely populated core of San Diego to the south, life is a bit slower in these towns. Here, surfing culture has thrived for decades.

But it's not all surfing, all the time. The best hiking opportunities along the North County coastal area center on the immediate coastline, especially along select stretches of sandy beach and also along the margins of several coastal lagoons.

For casual hikers, these venues nearly always offer easy walking and mild—even cool—weather conditions. On the beach itself, there's plenty of surfing talent to ogle, and alongside the lagoons a wide variety of birds will capture your attention.

One caveat: Warm summer weekends may bring throngs of beachgoers to the coastline, making parking a severe challenge. The solution, of course, is to get there early or wait until late afternoon.

◘ ◘ ◘

Hosp Grove

Trailhead Location: North Carlsbad, just inland from the coast

Trail Use: Hiking, running, dog walking

Distance & Configuration: 1.5-mile loop when including all trailhead spurs

Elevation Range: From near sea level to 185'

Facilities: Water, picnic tables, restrooms, and playground structures near the trailhead; The Shoppes at Carlsbad lie 0.5 mile east.

Highlights: Easy hiking, shade-giving eucalyptus trees, and migrating monarch butterflies

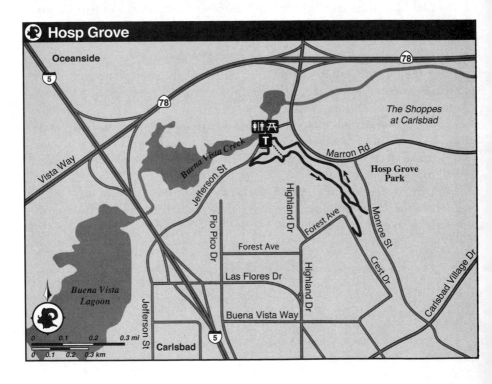

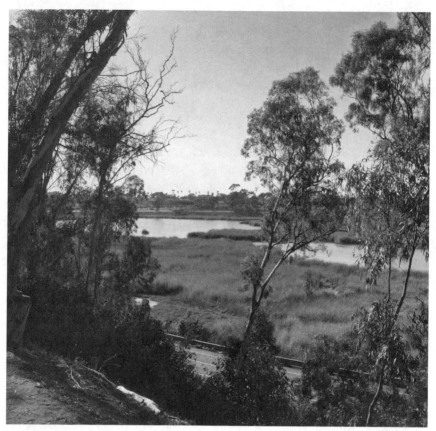

Buena Vista Lagoon

DESCRIPTION

For better or worse, eucalyptus trees from Australia have become a major component of San Diego County's contemporary urban forest. More than a century ago, entrepreneurs planted tall varieties of eucalyptus all over San Diego County (and in other parts of California) in a misguided effort to produce wood for railroad ties. These trees largely escaped the ax after people discovered that eucalyptus wood cracks and splits too easily for use as lumber. Thus, young and old eucalyptus trees still drape some hillsides just east of I-5 and above Buena Vista Lagoon in Carlsbad, at a place called Hosp Grove. Within Hosp Grove, the city of Carlsbad maintains a small nature park and trail system, providing a patch of serenity in an otherwise busy corner of North County.

THE ROUTE

You'll find the Hosp Grove Trail rising on the slope behind the park's tot play area. Alternatively, heading west from the small Jefferson Street parking lot (Trailhead 1 sign), you can ascend gradually to a view of Buena Vista Lagoon just above the first switchback. From several spots along this section of trail, you can peer over the tall, obscuring vegetation on the shoreline. Bring along binoculars—or, better yet, a spotting telescope—to observe the birdlife below.

The main Hosp Grove Trail goes left from the top of the short hill, contouring southeast, quite high along a steep slope, through the eucalyptus forest. Not much grows here other than eucalyptus because the leaf litter from these trees poisons nearly every other type of plant. Eucalyptus branches, though, are attractive to monarch butterflies. This colorful species migrates from summer homes in the Sierra Nevada and the Rocky Mountains, arriving at Hosp Grove and about two dozen other sites around San Diego County in November.

After less than 0.5 mile, the main Hosp Grove Trail descends, turns sharply left, and returns to Hosp Grove Park alongside city streets: first Monroe Street, and then Marron Road. If you choose the path to the right at this junction, you will pass a switchback and reach the high point of the grove along Crest Drive. Situated near the Trailhead 6 sign is a rope and board swing enticingly suspended from a stout eucalyptus that may tempt your inner child. Returning back down the way you just came, go right at the first fork and continue down toward the street in front of you. Just east of here, across Monroe Street, additional trails meander amid the eucalyptus trees overlooking The Shoppes at Carlsbad. Turn left on the path paralleling Monroe Street and follow it back to the parking area where you began your hike.

TO THE TRAILHEAD

GPS Coordinates: N33º 10.648'   W117º 20.501'

From the west, exit I-5 at Las Flores Drive (Exit 51A) in Carlsbad. Go west on Las Flores a short distance, then turn right on Jefferson Street. Proceed 0.6 mile to Hosp Grove Park on the right, opposite Buena Vista Lagoon.

From the east, exit CA 78 at Jefferson Street (Exit 1C), proceed south, and continue on Jefferson 0.7 mile to the Hosp Grove parking lot. Jefferson Street makes a hard right turn at 0.5 mile from the CA 78 exit, and the road that goes straight transitions into Marron Road. If you reach Monroe Street, turn around and go back 0.2 mile to make a left on Jefferson Street.

2 Guajome Regional Park

Trailhead Location: Oceanside

Trail Use: Hiking, running, biking, dog walking, horseback riding

Distance & Configuration: 4.0 miles of trails with multiple loops

Elevation Range: 100'–200'

Facilities: Restrooms and water at Main Entrance Picnic Area and Lower Entrance Picnic Area; playgrounds; developed campground (33 partial hookup sites)

Highlights: Cattail-rimmed Guajome Lake and secluded Upper Pond, freshwater marsh, nature trail, birding, overnight camping, QR Fit Trail

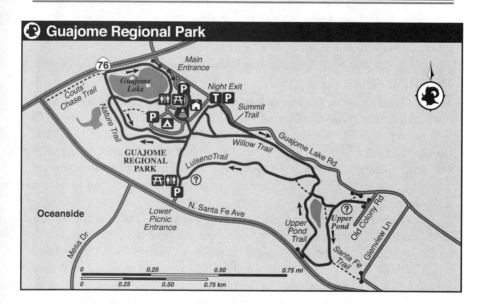

DESCRIPTION

Afternoon ocean breezes keep Guajome Regional Park temperate year-round, making it a popular destination for neighbors and visitors to engage in outdoors activities, including hiking, biking, or riding horseback on nearly 4 miles of trails that wind through and around this gentle coastal terrain. The park is home to a variety of native birds and animals and serves as an important rest stop for seasonal migrators. According to the park brochure, at least 186 species of birds have been recorded here.

Located 7 miles east of Oceanside and the ever-busy I-5, Guajome Regional Park features a deceptively natural setting that has been developed in various ways, going back to the California mission period. Originally inhabited by the native Luiseño Indians (so named by the padres of Mission San Luis Rey), this land was granted to two Luiseño brothers by the last governor of Mexican California in 1845. Ownership passed to several other parties before being gifted to Ysidora Bandini de Couts as a wedding present. Ysidora's husband, Cave Johnson Couts Sr., built Rancho Guajome Adobe, located 1 mile to the east. Rancho Guajome Adobe is a National Historic Landmark operated by San Diego County Parks and provides a wonderful venue for guided or self-guided trips back in time.

In the 1950s, owner Jerry Buteyn invested in several improvements, including constructing the lake and marsh area, planting palm trees, and terracing the land. The county purchased the land in 1970 to develop the current park and put finishing touches on the setting we enjoy here today.

So put on those hiking shoes, bring along water and a snack, and see for yourself what Guajome has to offer.

THE ROUTE

Six trailheads provide access to Guajome Regional Park, but only three have convenient parking. Two of these are adjacent to day-use areas ($3 fee)—one in the Main Entrance Picnic Area off Guajome Lake Road and the second in the Lower Picnic Entrance area off North Santa Fe Avenue. Day-use parking is 9:30 a.m.–sunset. A third hiking option, as described here, starts from the Night Exit just east of the main entrance on Guajome Lake Road.

Starting from the Night Exit, turn left on Summit Trail paralleling the road. Take in the expansive views looking out over the center portion of the park. Continue east and down a slight incline to merge with Upper Pond Trail/Willow Trail 0.2 mile from the start. The area on your right features a mix of grassland and riparian vegetation consisting of native and nonnative plants. This is an excellent area to watch for raptors, such as northern harriers and red-tailed hawks, impressively soaring or dropping low in search of prey. Bring along binoculars to appreciate their aerial skills. In another 0.25 mile, the trail intersects the Luiseno Trail heading to the right. Continue straight on Upper Pond Trail to a second intersection, the start of a loop path around Upper Pond. Cattails and reeds obscure the margins of Upper

Pond, providing protection and hunting opportunities for the resident critters. There are a couple of small access points around the loop. Proceed in either direction and return to the same point, then back to the Luiseno Trail junction, having traveled a little over 0.75 mile to complete the loop.

Returning to Luiseno Trail, turn left and follow it through the heart of Guajome Regional Park, coming out at the Lower Picnic Entrance in 0.6 mile. Along the way, you pass along marshy grasslands, palms, and a few relics of the irrigation system that helped create these wetlands. This is another great area for birding.

After pausing for lunch or a snack or enjoying playground time with children young and old, head back to the Luiseno Trail and proceed northerly on a wide path that crosses over small channels that bring water to the marshland in the westernmost section. Turn left in 0.125 mile to follow the Nature Trail or just beyond it on a path along the lower margins of the campground to reach Guajome Lake, 0.33 mile to the west. Once again, you can choose to go clockwise or counterclockwise around this 0.7-mile loop. The lake margins are less closed in than at Upper Pond, and several openings provide access for admiring the beauty of this oasis for humans and animals alike. Late afternoon lighting on the lake, as viewed from the west end, can be particularly attractive and a good excuse to have a camera with you.

Return to the Night Exit starting point via one of multiple footpaths from the Main Entrance Picnic Area or along Guajome Lake Road.

TO THE TRAILHEAD
GPS Coordinates: N33° 14.747'   W117° 16.210'

Exit I-5 at CA 76 (Exit 54A) in Oceanside. Drive 7.4 miles east and turn right onto Guajome Lake Road. The main entrance is 0.4 mile on the right. An automated ticket machine supplies day-use tickets for $3 per vehicle. The Night Exit trailhead is another 1,000 feet east of the main entrance, also on the right.

3 Batiquitos Lagoon

Trailhead Location: South Carlsbad, just inland from the coast

Trail Use: Hiking, running, dog walking

Distance & Configuration: 2.8-mile out-and-back

Elevation Range: Basically flat, just above sea level

Facilities: Water and restrooms at the start; the nature center at the trailhead is open daily, 9 a.m.–3 p.m.

Highlights: Fresh coastal breezes and one of the best bird-watching opportunities in San Diego County. Bring binoculars!

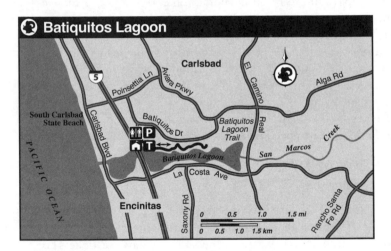

DESCRIPTION

Just beyond the placid north shoreline of Batiquitos Lagoon, white flecks of shell glint in the sunlight where the land begins to rise. Centuries ago, American Indians of this region gathered and consumed shellfish here. As generations of natives discarded the shell remains over thousands of years, their middens (refuse piles) grew in size and extent. Keep a sharp eye out, and you may see evidence of those middens today.

The Batiquitos Lagoon of prehistoric and early historic times lived up to its lagoon designation. Seawater surged in and out on the tides, alternately bathing and uncovering the low-lying, salt-tolerant vegetation, referred to as salt marsh habitat, an ecosystem of salt-tolerant vegetation increasingly threatened by coastal development throughout Southern California. In the 20th century, however, vast loads of soil loosened by agricultural activity and urban development on the lagoon's watersheds were flushed downstream during winter floods. Much of this silt dropped out of suspension near the lagoon's mouth, forming a plug that interfered with normal tidal flows. As a result, Batiquitos Lagoon lost its permanent connection to the ocean and became a stagnating, freshwater lake.

In a giant leap backward, or forward as the case may be, a massive dredging and lagoon restoration project in the 1990s converted the body of water back into a functioning estuary. Millions of cubic yards of sand were dredged from the lagoon's bottom and entrance channel and deposited on

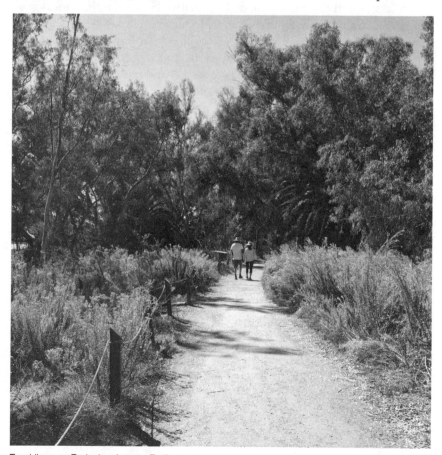

Two hikers on Batiquitos Lagoon Trail

nearby beaches or piled up along the lagoon shoreline to provide nesting sites for least terns and western snowy plovers.

Today, you may meander along a delightful trail on the restored lagoon's north shoreline. For the best bird-watching results, arrive here during early morning or late afternoon, when resident shorebirds and migrating visitors are most active. This also makes a good spot to cool off during one of San Diego's rare summer or autumn heat waves, when temperatures can reach into the 90s.

THE ROUTE

Starting from the Gabbiano Lane trailhead, head eastward on the main trail. The nearly level pathway curls along the lagoon's north shore, where colorful interpretive panels provide informative background on local flora and fauna. Traffic noise from I-5, annoying at first, fades as you continue east and pass several small eucalyptus coppices. An iron fence separates a perfectly manicured golf course and upscale housing on your left from the wild assortment of native sage scrub vegetation and nonnative palms, eucalyptus, mustard, and fennel on the shoreline strip you're walking through. (Along the route four side trails lead north to small parking lots along Batiquitos Drive.)

At a point 1.4 miles from the start, the shoreline trail pulls left and goes under dense eucalyptus foliage. This is a fine resting or picnic spot, and also a good place to turn around and return to the trailhead.

TO THE TRAILHEAD

GPS Coordinates: N33° 5.617'   W117° 18.077'

Exit I-5 at Poinsettia Lane (Exit 45) in Carlsbad. Proceed east on Poinsettia 0.3 mile, and turn right on Batiquitos Drive. Continue 0.5 mile, and turn right on Gabbiano Lane, which leads directly to the Batiquitos Lagoon parking lot, nature center, and trailhead.

4 Swami's Beach

Trailhead Location: On Coast Highway 101, just south of downtown Encinitas

Trail Use: Hiking, running, and wading in the surf

Distance & Configuration: 2.9-mile out-and-back

Elevation Range: From sea level to 100' at clifftop

Facilities: Public restrooms and picnic tables at Swami's Park; plenty of beach-flavored eateries on Coast Highway 101, north of K Street

Highlights: Sheer cliffs and well-formed waves; ideal for surfing and beachcombing

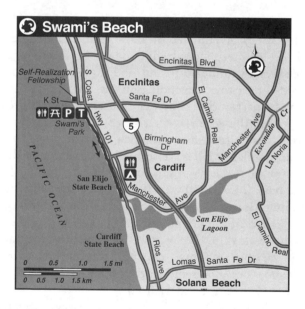

DESCRIPTION

The North County beach vibe finds its best expression in coastal Encinitas, where laid-back surfing and New Age cultures blend. Right below the high perch of the Asian-styled Self-Realization Fellowship (SRF) retreat, called Swami's in deference to founder Paramahansa Yogananda, lies one of San Diego County's most popular surfing spots. Just take it from the Beach

Boys, who referred to Swami's in their 1960s song "Surfin' USA." On most days throughout the year, you can view surfers in action or bobbing astride their boards just outside the breakers awaiting the next perfect wave. Bottlenose dolphins occasionally show up too, seemingly playing in the surf and sometimes even catching their own rides. Birds of many varieties—including gulls, terns, and shorebirds large and small, along with the ever-entertaining peeps (small sandpipers)—are likely to be present during a Swami's walk.

Our walk down the beach from Swami's Park, overlooking Swami's Beach, is flat and easy, with no more than a few cobbles here and there to trip you up. If you want, on the way down the beach or on the way back, you can ratchet up the exercise by climbing up and down several staircases. The staircases lead to the clifftop campgrounds of San Elijo State Beach. These sideways diversions involve little added horizontal distance and plenty of elevation gain and loss if you're game for it.

THE ROUTE

You begin the beach journey at pint-size Swami's Park. From the edge of the cliff, descend the 145 steep steps leading down the sheer slope to Swami's Beach, which is rocky to the north and sandy to the south. Simply head south on the wide or narrow (depending on the tide level) strip of sand that soon becomes a part of San Elijo State Beach. During extreme low-tide episodes in winter, the water level recedes 50–75 yards from the base of the sea bluffs, exposing sandstone reefs rich in marine life. This is less likely to happen in summer or fall because gentle wave action in those seasons tends to deposit a thicker layer of sand on the beach.

Even though the busy Coast Highway 101 lies atop the bluffs, you can't see it. The summertime sensual experience at the water's edge includes the soothing sound of the pounding surf, an ever-steady breeze out of the west caressing your skin, the spicy scent of salt-tinged air, and, of course, sunshine in variable amounts—depending on the cloud cover. (Take off your hiking shoes or sandals and let the foamy water lap around your feet and ankles to enhance this experience.)

As you proceed south, you will pass six separate stairways ascending the bluffs. Likely you'll spot some local runners scooting up and down—or down and up—these stairs for interval training. Some 1.4 miles into the beach walk, you reach the San Elijo Lagoon inlet, where tidal water flows in and out across the beach. This is a good spot to turn around and head back north. Consider checking out the clifftop campsites accessible from

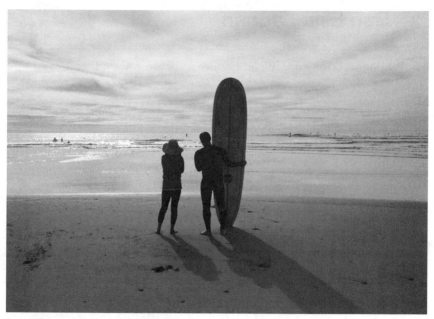

Big board dreamin' at San Elijo State Beach

each of the six staircases leading up from the beach. Public restrooms are also available here.

Before you return to your car, or perhaps at another time, consider visiting the SRF Meditation Gardens, overlooking the ocean at the west end of K Street (215 W. K St.). This serene spot is open to the public Tuesday–Saturday, 9 a.m.–5 p.m., and Sunday, 11 a.m.–5 p.m. There is no charge. (See encinitastemple.org.)

TO THE TRAILHEAD

GPS Coordinates: N33° 2.079'   W117° 17.521'

Exit I-5 at Encinitas Boulevard (Exit 42). Go west to South Coast Highway 101, make a left, and travel south past lettered streets (C, D, E, and so on) for 0.9 mile to K Street on the right. Find a curbside parking space on K Street, on the west side of 101, or just about anywhere within a reasonable distance of K Street. Parking along Third Street near J Street is typically a good option for busy times. If you're lucky (fat chance in the summer), you might find a parking space in the small lot at Swami's Park, which is on 101, one long block south of K Street.

5 San Elijo Lagoon

Trailhead Location: Inland from coast between Cardiff and Solana Beach

Trail Use: Hiking, running, dog walking

Distance & Configuration: Up to 4 miles out-and-back on East Basin paths and another 2 miles in West Basin, including Annie's Canyon Trail

Elevation Range: Sea level to 180' at the top of Annie's Canyon

Facilities: No facilities at the main trailheads; access to water and restrooms at the lagoon's nature center on the north shore

Highlights: Five plant communities thrive within a small elevation range; plenty of bird-watching opportunities; unique sandstone slot canyon

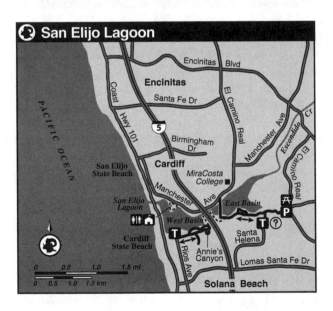

DESCRIPTION

A great blue heron ambles on stilt legs across the reed-fringed shallows, stabbing occasionally at subsurface morsels of food. Nearby, a willowy egret glides in for a perfect landing, scattering concentric ripples across the surface of the lagoon. Both species seem oblivious to binocular-toting humans who spy on them—from a comfortable distance.

A scene like this is repeated almost daily at San Elijo Lagoon, centerpiece of the San Elijo Lagoon Ecological Preserve, on public lands jointly administered by the San Elijo Lagoon Conservancy, County of San Diego Parks and Recreation Department, and California Department of Fish and Wildlife.

West of I-5, in the West Basin part of the lagoon, high tides wash over mudflats and mats of salt-tolerant vegetation. Because of the habitat diversity, you can see a dozen kinds of shorebirds on a typical day. In fact, some 300 bird species have been spotted in and around the lagoon over a period of years, and about 300 species of plants have been identified here. In addition to providing world-class birding opportunities, the West Basin also features one of San Diego's newest hiking venues, Annie's Canyon Trail, which opened in June 2016 following extensive restoration work. Annie's Canyon is a truly special place featuring towering sandstone walls; nooks and crannies that host shade-loving native plants; and thrilling, sloping, body-tight squeezes to pass through a rare coastal slot canyon.

The East Basin portion of the lagoon, east of I-5, is a freshwater marsh, supported by runoff from Escondido Creek and La Orilla Creek. Like its western counterpart but typically less visited, the East Basin provides expansive marshland views and great birding of its own.

THE ROUTE

Two significant hiking routes take you along the shores of San Elijo Lagoon. From the Rios Avenue trailhead, you can follow beautiful paths that meander along the West Basin's south shore. You will stroll by coastal sage scrub vegetation, which looks bright green in winter and spring and drab in summer and fall. You will also walk through groves of eucalyptus and other nonnative trees. Eroded sandstone bluffs half-hidden behind a screen of vegetation provide an impressive backdrop for the placid lagoon. Annie's Canyon Trail starts approximately 0.5 mile from the trailhead along the southern section of the main loop trail. Turn right and continue south about 70 yards to a signed junction with arrows. The right fork ascends Annie's Canyon in a counterclockwise loop, steep and narrow in places, and eventually climbs out via a steel ladder through colorful bands of sandstone to reach the viewpoint, followed by a descent on an open and more gradual trail leading back to the junction. Going left reverses this route to the viewpoint. The inner canyon is marked as a one-way loop at the junction sign. Descending from the viewpoint should be avoided during busy periods as there is little room for one person to negotiate the narrowest sections, let alone space to pass another party going the opposite way. Inside the canyon is like visiting another world. Fanciful fingertips (*Dudleya edulis*) sprout from vertical walls. Scramble up a south-facing cave in the middle upper section for a great view of the inaccessible upper reaches due south. Watch your step, though, as the footing can be slippery here even when wearing hiking boots.

After descending from the viewpoint and returning to the main trail, continue to the right another 0.1 mile where you are approaching the embankment of ever-busy I-5. Though you could turn back here and return to the Rios Avenue trailhead, there is a better option. Take a small trail north, then turn left at the first junction and follow the edge of the lagoon back to the west. This is a great trail for observing ducks and wading birds, especially if you brought along binoculars.

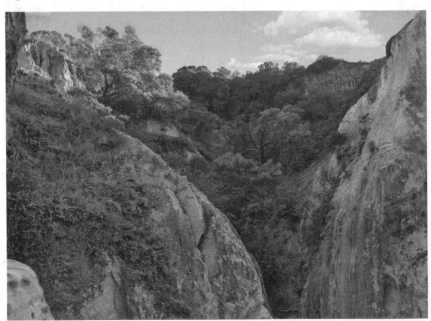

Annie's Canyon

The second significant hike is an exploration of the lagoon's East Basin (east of I-5) starting from the south via one of four neighborhood trailheads. A recommended route enters from the end of Santa Helena. After passing an information kiosk, the trail descends gradually on a service road to an intersection with an east-west trail. Turn right to pass through forested stretches of pine and eucalyptus, terminating in 0.5 mile at El Camino Real and the San Orilla trailhead. There is a small parking lot here and picnic tables.

Reverse your route to return to the intersection with the service road, then continue west to reach the best vistas of East Basin. Benches are strategically placed at several vantage points. As you approach I-5 with a few more ups and downs over eroded hills, you come to a T. Turn right to traverse the top of a flood-control dike leading north to the Manchester Avenue pedestrian gate. The dike helps maintain these wetlands and provides great access for up close birding. Turn around at this point to return to Santa Helena by the same route.

The trail connection between the East and West Basins is closed due to highway improvements and is not expected to reopen until 2021, when the project is complete.

Note: If you don't have much time, you may want to take the short, looping interpretive trail that originates from the San Elijo Lagoon Nature Center on Manchester Avenue, 0.5 mile west of I-5. You'll enjoy direct access to the north shore of West Basin. It's the place to go not for exercise, but rather (arguably) for the best chance to see the greatest variety of birds.

TO THE TRAILHEAD
GPS Trailhead Coordinates:
Rios Avenue Trailhead: N33° 0.223'   W117° 16.334'
Santa Helena Trailhead: N33° 0.433'   W117° 14.863'

To get to the Rios Avenue trailhead, exit I-5 at Lomas Santa Fe Drive (Exit 37) in Solana Beach. Go west 0.8 mile to Rios Avenue, turn right, and continue 0.8 mile north to the end of Rios Avenue and the Rios Avenue trailhead.

To get to the Santa Helena trailhead, exit I-5 at Lomas Santa Fe Drive (Exit 37) in Solana Beach. Go east on Lomas Santa Fe then immediately turn left on Santa Helena. Follow Santa Helena 1.5 miles until it ends at the trailhead.

6 Del Mar Crest & Beach

Trailhead Location: Del Mar

Trail Use: Hiking, running

Distance & Configuration: 5-mile loop

Elevation Range: Sea level to 360'

Facilities: None at the trailhead; water, restaurants, and small shopping plazas in Del Mar en route within the first 2 miles; water and restrooms at Powerhouse Park and Torrey Pines State Beach

Highlights: Pine-dotted canyon vistas and a long stretch of isolated beach

DESCRIPTION

Combining canyon, crest, and sandy strand, this loop hike touches on every natural landscape that the woodsy community of Del Mar has to offer. The tide line scenery along the route is some of the best in San Diego County. Be aware, though, that high tides, particularly in winter, can flood the beach segment of the route. Check tide tables first if you expect to travel along the sand. If the tides do flood the beach, there is a not-as-pleasant alternate route to consider and another choice *not* to consider (see page 31).

THE ROUTE

Start off at the north end of Del Mar Scenic Parkway, where a sign announces that you are entering the Torrey Pines State Natural Reserve Extension, an annex of the main Torrey Pines State Natural Reserve, which lies south (Hike 19, page 72). Pets are strictly prohibited in the extension ahead and on Torrey Pines State Beach. Dogs are seasonally allowed on leash on Del Mar Beach, except for summer months, between Powerhouse Park and the Torrey Pines State Beach boundary near Sixth Street. Follow the bottom of the ravine on what is signed as TRAIL B.

A number of large Torrey pines grace the reserve extension area, their long needles in bundles of five illustrating their identity. The natural range of the Torrey pine, one of the rarest pines in the world, is restricted to the coastal bluffs near Del Mar, Santa Rosa Island, and Lompoc. If you want

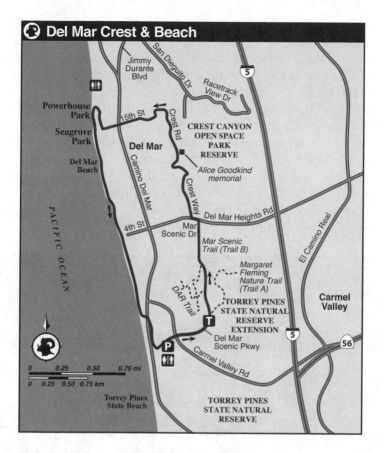

Del Mar Crest & Beach

(Map labels)

Jimmy Durante Blvd
San Dieguito Dr
Racetrack View Dr
5
Powerhouse Park
15th St
Crest Rd
CREST CANYON OPEN SPACE PARK RESERVE
Seagrove Park
Del Mar
Alice Goodkind memorial
Del Mar Beach
Camino Del Mar
Crest Way
Del Mar Heights Rd
El Camino Real
PACIFIC OCEAN
4th St
Mar Scenic Dr
Mar Scenic Trail (Trail B)
Margaret Fleming Nature Trail (Trail A)
DAR Trail
TORREY PINES STATE NATURAL RESERVE EXTENSION
Carmel Valley
T
Del Mar Scenic Pkwy
5
56
P
Carmel Valley Rd
0   0.25   0.50   0.75 mi
0   0.25   0.50   0.75 km
Torrey Pines State Beach
TORREY PINES STATE NATURAL RESERVE

to see more of these beautiful trees, consider a side excursion on the short Daughters of the American Revolution (DAR) Trail, branching to the left of Trail B. Another option is to take Trail A, a right fork near the starting point. This lesser-traveled route is the Margaret Fleming Nature Trail, a 1.3-mile out-and-back path named for the wife of Guy Fleming, the park's first custodian, who began in that capacity back in 1921. Guy and Margaret raised their family near the historic lodge that now serves as park head-quarters. Her husband's contributions are commemorated with a plaque on the scenic Guy Fleming Trail, the northernmost of the paths described in Hike 19, Torrey Pines State Natural Reserve. How fitting to have trails named for this pioneering Torrey Pines couple.

Sticking with the straight-and-narrow Trail B, you arrive after only 0.5 mile at the dead end of Mar Scenic Drive. Keep straight (north) for two blocks, turn left on busy Del Mar Heights Road, and go one short block to reach a traffic signal 0.7 mile into the hike. Use it to cross Del Mar Heights Road and pick up Crest Way, heading north. Crest Way (signed as Crest Road as you continue north) follows the rim of what is called Crest Canyon, a patch of open space on the right harboring picturesque sandstone formations and several large native Torrey pines. Watch for birds of prey wheeling overhead, taking advantage of the thermals.

Crest Road ahead is narrow and without sidewalks. Despite its frequent speed bumps intended to calm traffic, you will need to be vigilant of cars. However, Crest Road traverses one of Del Mar's most exclusive residential neighborhoods, so there's plenty of architectural and floral eye candy to look at. The landscaping includes outsize Torrey pines, which owe their height and girth here to the modern-day miracle of irrigation.

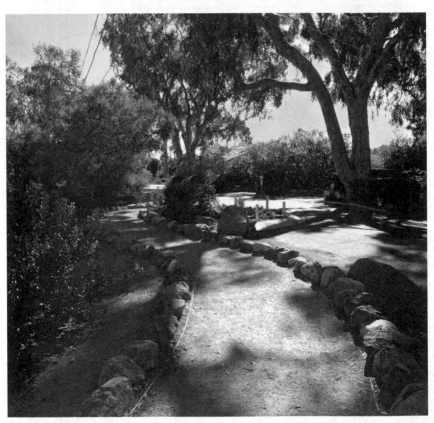

Alice Goodkind memorial

At 1.4 miles into the hike and just past Amphitheater Drive, you will pass a small area featuring stone benches that face eastward out over Crest Canyon. This attractive oasis is dedicated to Alice Goodkind, a Del Mar resident, musician, writer, and volunteer activist who supported protection for a number of natural spaces in the area. Just beyond the Goodkind memorial, continue north another 0.25 mile and make a sharp left from Crest Road onto 15th Street. You descend quickly to Camino Del Mar, which is the name of Pacific Coast Highway 101 as it traverses the city of Del Mar. Care for a cup of coffee or other refreshment here? There are lots of choices.

After your break, continue downhill to the adjacent Seagrove and Powerhouse Parks (2.5 miles from the start), where you cross the railroad tracks and gain access to the beach. Now go south along the coastline. Low tides are perfect for the 1.6-mile-long straight stretch of sand-walking that lies ahead. If the beach is flooded by high tide or has unusually heavy surf, you may walk along Camino Del Mar as you continue south.

Note: As another alternative, some walkers and runners follow the railroad tracks on the bluff overlooking the beach. However, every hour or so, passenger trains whoosh along the rail corridor, often with little warning. Therefore, this guidebook strongly recommends that under no circumstances should you consider this illegal and unsafe route.

The stretch of beach below the bluffs is terrific, with the sounds of only a passing train or a happy, barking dog every now and again: this is a popular (and rare) instance of a San Diego–area beach being open to *leashed* dogs.

At a bit over 4 miles into the hike, turn inland under the Camino Del Mar Bridge to reach a large parking lot for Torrey Pines State Beach. Walk out to the parking lot entrance on Carmel Valley Road, cross over to the other side, and keep going up the sidewalk of Del Mar Scenic Parkway. Walk all the way to the end of the street to your parked car.

TO THE TRAILHEAD
GPS Coordinates: N32° 56.299'   W117° 15.164'

Exit I-5 at Carmel Valley Road (Exit 33) in Del Mar. Drive 1.1 miles west to Del Mar Scenic Parkway on the right, directly across from the Torrey Pines State Beach entrance. Proceed to the end of that street, where curbside parking is available.

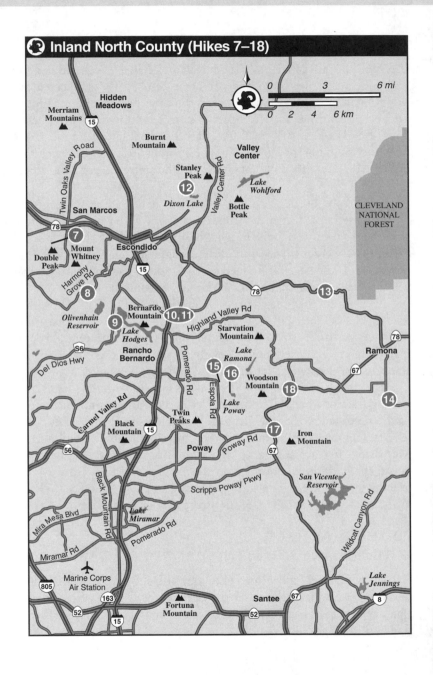

Inland North County (Hikes 7–18)

Merriam Mountains

Hidden Meadows

15

Burnt Mountain

Twin Oaks Valley Road

Valley Center

Stanley Peak

12

Dixon Lake

Valley Center Rd

Lake Wohlford

Bottle Peak

CLEVELAND NATIONAL FOREST

San Marcos

78

7

Escondido

Double Peak

Mount Whitney

Harmony Grove Rd

15

8

78

13

Olivenhain Reservoir

9

Bernardo Mountain

10,11

Highland Valley Rd

Lake Hodges

Starvation Mountain

78

S6

Rancho Bernardo

Ramona

Del Dios Hwy

Pomerado Rd

Lake Ramona

67

Carmel Valley Rd

15

Espola Rd

16

Woodson Mountain

18

14

Twin Peaks

Lake Poway

Black Mountain

56

Poway

17

Iron Mountain

67

Poway Rd

Scripps Poway Pkwy

San Vicente Reservoir

Black Mountain Rd

Wildcat Canyon Rd

Mira Mesa Blvd

Lake Miramar

Pomerado Rd

Miramar Rd

Lake Jennings

805

Marine Corps Air Station

163

52

15

Fortuna Mountain

Santee

67

52

8

0   3   6 mi

0   2   4   6 km

INLAND NORTH COUNTY

A wrinkled landscape of rock-ribbed hills, small mountains, and gently sloping valleys characterizes the inland North County region. From such quintessentially suburban communities as San Marcos, Escondido, Rancho Bernardo, and Poway in the west, the land steadily rises east toward the even more corrugated interior rural landscape forming the foothills of San Diego County's major massifs—the Palomar, Cuyamaca, and Laguna Mountains.

The inland suburban climate is not as benign as that along the coastline. Summer daytime temperatures often rise into the 90s, and wintertime frost occasionally dusts the valleys. Farther inland, in the rural zone around the community of Ramona, summer highs sometimes exceed 100°F. While these temperatures are not remarkably extreme for many parts of the country, it is worth noting that, around here in general, the coming of the sun-splashed summer does not equate to great hiking. It is simply too hot and too dry. Not until October or November do those conditions abate. If you must hike during these potentially scorching months, confine your explorations to early morning or late afternoon and early evening.

When you do hike here, the highly topographical nature of inland North County's landscape ensures that you will be treated to beautiful and often breathtaking vistas. Whether you are cradled in the bottom of a valley or have reached the crest of a peak, the view will almost never disappoint.

Be forewarned that drinking water is scarce along trails that thread through inland North County. The same trails also gain and lose significant amounts of elevation, which only increases the effort of those who hike them. So for reasons of both safety and comfort, hikers are strongly encouraged to take along plenty of water, especially when the weather is warm.

7 Double Peak

Trailhead Location: San Marcos, near California State University

Trail Use: Hiking, running, dog walking, mountain biking, horseback riding

Distance & Configuration: 4.6-mile out-and-back

Elevation Range: 670' at the start to 1,644' at the peak

Facilities: Water and restrooms at the start and on the summit of Double Peak

Highlights: Panoramic views of the entire inland North County area, along with an ocean vista from the top

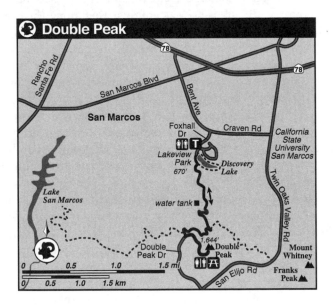

DESCRIPTION

South of the spreading suburbs that cluster along CA 78, a scruffy ridge-line scrapes the southern sky. Topographic maps note the obscure names of its various high points: Cerro de las Posas, Double Peak, Franks Peak, and Mount Whitney (not *that* Whitney but still the highest of the group). Double Peak, our destination on this hike, is the most hiker-friendly. Its summit lies within a City of San Marcos regional/interpretive park that takes full advantage of the peak's panoramic view. When the park was completed in 2009, it became possible to drive all the way to the summit from the San Elijo Hills housing development on the south side. Our chosen route, however, goes up Double Peak's mostly undeveloped north slope and capitalizes on a roughly 1,000-foot elevation change. That is appealing, of course, only if you're amenable to a bit of vigorous exercise.

THE ROUTE

You begin at Lakeview Park next to a small reservoir called Discovery Lake. A flat 0.8-mile trail, popular with everyone from runners to parents pushing strollers, loops around the lake. Our way to Double Peak, though, takes you across the lake's dam to a paved, traffic-free maintenance road heading south and sharply up a hillside through chaparral vegetation. Numbered white trail signs are located at key points all the way up, including at trail junctions and street crossings. Simply head in the direction of the red arrows labeled DOUBLE PEAK TRAIL. Soon, you go into and then out of a hillside residential development. Just continue uphill toward a large, hillside water tank. Just shy of the tank, turn left on a fenced dirt path and climb very steeply through chaparral nicely recovering from the last big fire in 1996. North-slope vegetation such as this requires about 40 years of growth to reach a climax stage, and this stand is on its way.

At the next trail intersection—1.1 miles from the start and identified with one of the Double Peak Trail signs and a low-to-the-ground, circular brass plaque labeled SAN ELIJO HILLS 10K LOOP START—turn sharply right and continue climbing more moderately until you reach a multiuse recreation path running along the ridgeline. Make a left there (going southeast), and you will soon come to Double Peak Drive, which at this point is curling up from the San Elijo Hills housing development. Simply get on the sidewalk and continue walking steeply uphill until you reach Double Peak Park's parking lot.

Scattered eucalyptus trees and olive trees, relics from an old homesite, dot the summit itself, and now those trees have been joined by picnic tables thoughtfully placed to frame the spectacular view. At the very top, a free-to-use swiveling telescope that rotates 360 degrees is affixed to the center of a concrete pad and can be used for sighting key landmarks. The extent of the view depends on the season, with late fall and winter months generally providing the greatest atmospheric transparency. Even on an average day, you can at least glimpse Southern California's highest mountain ranges (the San Gabriels, San Bernardinos, and San Jacintos) in the north and the shining

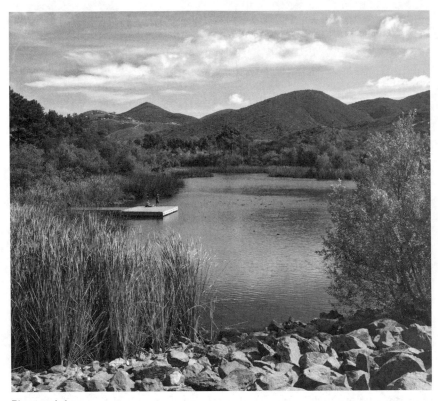

Discovery Lake

Pacific Ocean to the west and southwest. On days of exceptional atmospheric clarity, add to that list Santa Catalina Island offshore from Orange and Los Angeles Counties and the Coronado Islands off the northern Baja coast. At this point you can retrace your steps back to the trailhead.

TO THE TRAILHEAD
GPS Coordinates: N33° 7.477'   W117° 10.737'

Exit CA 78 at Twin Oaks Valley Road (which ultimately becomes San Elijo Road, but you won't go that far) in San Marcos (Exit 13). Turn south and proceed 0.8 mile to Craven Road. Turn right on Craven and continue 0.7 mile to Foxhall Drive. Turn left on Foxhall and proceed to the end of the road and into the parking lot for Lakeview Park and Discovery Lake.

8 Elfin Forest Recreational Reserve

Trailhead Location: East of Escondido, near the community of Elfin Forest

Trail Use: Hiking, mountain biking, dog walking, running, horseback riding

Distance & Configuration: 7.2-mile balloon

Elevation Range: 500' at the start to 1,260'

Facilities: Water and restrooms at the trailhead and at Ridgetop Picnic Area; trailhead also has a small interpretive center

Highlights: Spacious views of inland North County, the ocean, and distant mountains

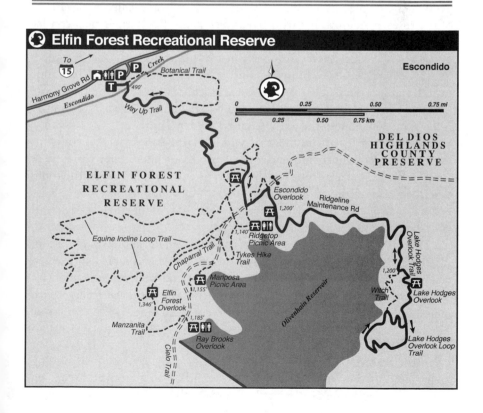

Elfin Forest Recreational Reserve

DESCRIPTION

The 784-acre Elfin Forest Recreational Reserve serves two purposes: water management and recreation. The Olivenhain Dam and Reservoir within the reserve holds nearly 8 billion gallons of water (24,000 acre-feet), providing an extra, temporary supply for the San Diego region in case an earthquake severs or damages aqueducts that transport water from Northern California. This capacity is estimated to be enough to meet the needs of 192,000 people for a year. The water-storage scheme also helps regulate the local demand for electricity. At times of peak electrical energy usage, water released from Olivenhain and falling toward Lake Hodges below generates supplemental electricity. During periods of lesser demand, often at night, water in Lake Hodges can be pumped back up the hill to replenish the reservoir.

The recreational component of Elfin Forest Recreational Reserve and its 11 miles of trails cater to all self-propelled travelers (hikers, runners, equestrians, and mountain bikers) and are uncommonly friendly toward pet owners. At present, on weekdays only, and only at the upper elevations of the reserve, dog owners who have voice control over their pets can let them off leash. *On weekends, dogs must be leashed.*

For small kids, there are short, nearly flat trails near the entrance, where Escondido Creek murmurs and splashes over boulders. The mile-long Botanical Trail, also near the entrance, features interpretive posts keyed to a leaflet. Ambitious hikers and bikers, though, must travel up the hill on the only route—the aptly named Way Up Trail.

They can fashion a number of wide-ranging loops, several miles in length, out of the intricate network of old roads and newer singletrack trails in the upland area south of the reserve's entrance. However, the route described here features the best views of both Olivenhain and Hodges Reservoirs. It also offers the most comprehensive vistas of the hills, valleys, and cities near and far.

As this challenging route almost constantly gains and loses elevation, you'll want to start the hike with a full water bottle and replenish it when you reach the Ridgetop Picnic Area on the out-and-back route segments.

Note: Expect to share this and most other routes in the reserve with mountain bikers, as they are welcome and common here.

THE ROUTE

From the reserve parking lot (open at 8 a.m. each day; seasonal closing hours are posted), cross Escondido Creek and begin a crooked ascent on the Way Up Trail. The canyon wall you are climbing is studded with tooth-like rock outcrops and dripping with thick, junglelike growths of chaparral.

As you may have guessed, the small community of Elfin Forest just west of here and the reserve itself are named after the local chaparral vegetation known as elfin forest. Until late in the spring, this cool, north-facing canyon wall also retains its spring-green grass and exhibits showy clusters of red monkey flower and nightshade.

The Ridgetop Picnic Area, with portable restrooms and drinking water, comes into view after 1.5 miles and about 700 feet of climbing. You're now on a rolling plateau, and the reservoir lies just ahead. Right before reaching the picnic area, you'll cross the unpaved Ridgeline Maintenance Road. After filling your water bottle, head east (uphill) on that road, and then make a right turn to curl downward past Escondido Overlook (another picnic site). The maintenance road continues east—as do you—along Olivenhain Reservoir's shoreline on a sometimes uphill, sometimes downhill course. Your gaze takes in the whole of the reservoir, its surface reflecting whatever color the sky happens to be at that time. On clear, blue-sky mornings, when the reservoir is filled to the brim, the azure surface is reminiscent of an enormous swimming pool with a vanishing edge at the dam on the far side.

At about 2.33 miles into the hike, the road narrows and becomes the Lake Hodges Overlook Trail. You dip sharply to reach the reservoir's shoreline and then climb abruptly back, eventually reaching Lake Hodges Overlook, with its picnic table and an amazing view of sprawling Lake Hodges below. The Lake Hodges Overlook Loop Trail lies just ahead, and it's worth it to travel the extra 0.8-mile distance around its looping course. If you do, you get to view the placid waters of Olivenhain Reservoir from different perspectives than before.

Whether you've taken the 1-mile add-on or not, you will begin your return hike from the Lake Hodges Overlook, going back the way you came, negotiating the same ups and downs, only in reverse order.

TO THE TRAILHEAD
GPS Coordinates: N33° 5.186'   W117° 8.716'

Exit I-15 at Ninth Avenue (Exit 30) in Escondido. Head west and proceed 0.2 mile. Turn left here, so as to remain on Ninth Avenue. (Auto Park Way continues straight ahead.) Continue 0.6 mile west on Ninth Avenue to a forced left turn onto Hale Avenue. Go 0.3 mile south on Hale, and turn right on Harmony Grove Road. Go 0.3 mile west and turn sharply left to remain on Harmony Grove Road. After another 0.4 mile, you must turn left again to remain on Harmony Grove Road, which becomes a rural byway at this point. Continue 3 miles to the Elfin Forest Recreational Reserve entrance on the left, near mile marker 6 on Harmony Grove Road.

9 Del Dios Gorge

Trailhead Location: Between Rancho Santa Fe and Escondido

Trail Use: Hiking, mountain biking, dog walking, horseback riding, running

Distance & Configuration: 6.4-mile out-and-back

Elevation Range: 410' down to 140' (river crossing)

Facilities: Water and portable restroom at the trailhead; restaurant across the street

Highlights: The historic Lake Hodges Dam and (rarely) rushing water down the gorge; riparian habitat

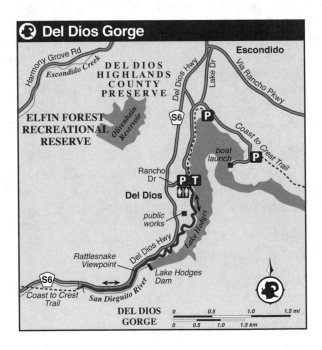

DESCRIPTION

On its roughly 50-mile course from the mountain crest near Julian to the beach at Del Mar, the combined Santa Ysabel Creek/San Dieguito River courses through several steep and narrow canyons. The lowest of these, the Del Dios Gorge, is partly inundated by Lake Hodges, a reservoir whose concrete-arch dam began to impound the waters of the San Dieguito River in 1918. Below that dam today, a steep section of the gorge remains in evidence. A section of the Coast to Crest Trail, which will one day stretch the entire length of the San Dieguito River and its main tributary, Santa Ysabel Creek, threads its way right down the gorge.

The best time by far to visit Del Dios Gorge is during winter—better yet if that winter season features above-average rainfall. Every few years, Lake Hodges overflows its spillway, adjacent to the dam. Under the right circumstances, the resulting spray can create a rainbow. Most of the time, because of the dry climate, there's no spillage from the reservoir, and water in the gorge slides gently by or gathers in algae-rich pools.

THE ROUTE

From the trailhead, follow the narrow, beaten-down path that swings right, parallel to the shore of Lake Hodges in the direction of the dam. Some mild ups and downs follow, with frequent views of the water below. At one point, you pass a large public works complex on the right. It houses electric pumps and generators that regulate the flow of water between Lake Hodges and the Olivenhain Reservoir, unseen on the high ridge above.

Nearly 2 miles into the hike, you reach a point alongside the nearly century-old concrete Lake Hodges Dam. Early on, the dam developed troublesome cracks, but by 1937 (following the devastating Long Beach earthquake of 1933), the dam had been strongly reinforced. Other than some painted-over graffiti, the dam retains its old-world architectural charm.

Just beyond the dam, the trail pulls right alongside Del Dios Highway. Soon, you turn abruptly left and descend toward the bottom of the gorge on an unpaved service road, doubling as the trail route. Notice the remnants of a flume that formerly connected Lake Hodges to a smaller storage facility, San Dieguito Reservoir, some 4 miles away.

At a switchback shortly after passing the service road pedestrian gate, an unusual pipe scope has been installed at Rattlesnake Viewpoint (so named because the stonework here was constructed in the shape of a rattlesnake). The pipe scope is accompanied with instructions for how to sight key features of the dam. Another interpretive sign provides a short history and features photographs associated with dam construction and its early years of operation. As you continue downhill and downstream, there's never a point where the noise from nearby Del Dios Highway isn't apparent, but at least you can admire the steeply rising far wall of the gorge and the scattered willows, oaks, and granite outcrops down along the river-bed. Restoration efforts are continuing, which will ultimately improve the habitat alongside the river, encourage the growth of native vegetation, and provide better foraging and nesting for birds.

At 3.2 miles from the start, the trail swings sharply left and crosses the San Dieguito River on an elaborate iron footbridge. The trail continues downcanyon from here another 1.2 miles before reaching the Santa Fe Valley Staging Area off Bing Crosby Boulevard, and then another 1.9 miles with steep switchbacks to a turnaround point in Santa Fe Valley near Lusardi Creek. Further travel on this trail in progress will someday allow you to walk all the way out to the beach at Del Mar, but our hike ends here at the bridge. Return the same way you came.

TO THE TRAILHEAD
GPS Coordinates: N33° 3.769'   W117° 7.182'

Exit I-15 at Via Rancho Parkway (Exit 27). Drive west on Via Rancho 3.5 miles, turn left at the Del Dios Highway traffic light, go 2 miles farther to Rancho Drive (traffic light), and turn left again. Rancho Drive goes downhill 0.3 mile to a San Dieguito River Park trailhead and staging area on the right. The famed Hernandez' Hide-Away biker bar/restaurant lies across the street from the trailhead.

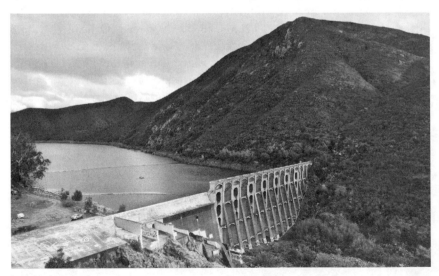

Lake Hodges Dam

10 Bernardo Mountain

Trailhead Location: South Escondido

Trail Use: Hiking, running, mountain biking, dog walking, birding

Distance & Configuration: 7.2-mile out-and-back

Elevation Range: 330' at the start to 1,150' at the summit

Facilities: Water and portable restroom at the trailhead and north end of the pedestrian bridge; myriad facilities at the giant North County Fair shopping center, 0.5 mile north of the trailhead

Highlights: A summit view encompassing Lake Hodges, plus valleys and mountains as far as the eye can see

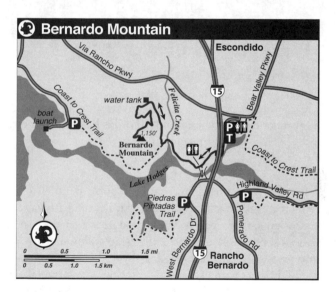

DESCRIPTION

The massive bulk of Bernardo Mountain rises from the north shoreline of Lake Hodges, almost like a smooth-sided pyramid. The summit area of the mountain was purchased for inclusion in the San Dieguito River Park in 2002, and that gave public access for hikers and bikers. The park, designed to preserve as much of nature as possible within the San Dieguito River/

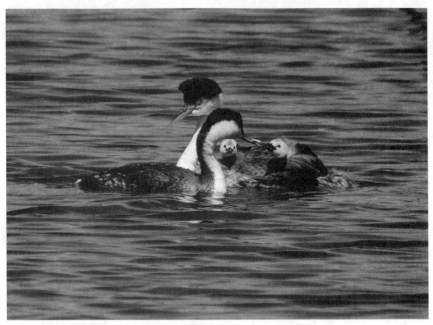

A grebe feeds fish to its babies on its mate's back.

Santa Ysabel Creek watershed, stretches about 50 miles between the coast-line at Del Mar and Volcan Mountain near Julian.

THE ROUTE

Start from the Sunset Drive trailhead by heading south, parallel to I-15, initially on a wide concrete walkway. After about 0.4 mile, the pathway turns sharply right and passes under the freeway bridge that goes over the east arm of Lake Hodges. You'll soon hook up with a dirt trail following the lake's north shoreline, going west. A short distance later, you'll come to the north end of an elaborate footbridge, completed in 2009, that spans the lake and runs parallel to the freeway. The David Kreitzer Lake Hodges Bicycle Pedes-trian Bridge is not a suspension bridge but rather a stressed ribbon bridge, a design selected to minimize its visual impact; 87 panels of 16-inch-thick, 12-foot-wide concrete decking constitutes the "ribbon" that is placed on top of tensioned steel cables stretching between anchors at each end. At 990 feet total length and 330 feet between supports, the Lake Hodges Bridge is the longest of this type in the world. If you want to make a short, optional side trip, cross the bridge and then return to this route.

Another feature of the east end of Lake Hodges, at least during wet winters, are the large numbers of western grebes that can be observed in their annual courtship ritual when pairs and threesomes rush across the water in synchronized choreography. This is just one example of why Lake Hodges was nominated by the Palomar Audubon Society as an Important Bird Area and in 1999 was the first site in California to hold a formal ceremony recognizing it as a Globally Important Bird Area. In addition to the aforementioned grebes and a sizable number of threatened California gnatcatchers, more than 200 different species of resident or migrating birds have been recorded here.

At 1.6 miles into your trip, you cross Felicita Creek, a small perennial brook deeply shaded by coast live oaks, western sycamores, and other native water-loving vegetation, as well as opportunistic invasive plants such as fan palms and date palms. After the creek crossing, make a right on the first available singletrack trail, marked with a sign, and head north toward Bernardo's summit.

You ascend gradually at first through scrubby chaparral vegetation, with the oaks and sycamores of Felicita Creek just below you on the right and Bernardo Mountain rising on the left. By about 2.5 miles, you've swung around to the north side of the mountain, where the views become more expansive. Much of what comes into view in the north are rural housing areas surrounding the city of Escondido. Stay left (uphill) at the next two trail intersections, always heading upward.

You continue ascending or contouring in a zigzag pattern, passing a large water tank at 3.2 miles and finally reaching the rocky summit at 3.6 miles. From this noble vantage point, you can clearly visualize the patchwork of city, suburbia, and wildland that inland North County has become. The white noise of traffic on I-15 wafts upward to you—but peering in certain other directions, you see little apparent human impact on the landscape. Westward, down the valley below Lake Hodges, a slice of Pacific Ocean is visible on clear days.

When you're ready to go, return the way you came.

TO THE TRAILHEAD
GPS Coordinates: N33° 3.973'   W117° 4.098'

Exit I-15 at Via Rancho Parkway (Exit 27) in south Escondido. Go east one long block to Sunset Drive. Turn right and drive 0.2 mile to the San Dieguito River Park trailhead and parking area.

11 Sikes Adobe and Mule Hill

Trailhead Location: South Escondido

Trail Use: Hiking, running, mountain biking, dog walking

Distance & Configuration: 2.6-mile out-and-back

Elevation Range: 330' at the start to 360'

Facilities: Water and portable restrooms at the trailhead; myriad facilities at the giant Westfield North County shopping center, 0.5 mile north of the trailhead

Highlights: Historic farmhouse and a Mexican-American War battle site

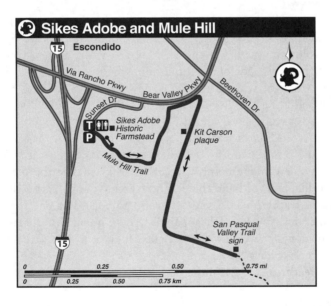

DESCRIPTION

This short, mostly level hike follows the Mule Hill Trail, a section of the Coast to Crest Trail administered as part of the San Dieguito River Park trail system. The park, designed to preserve as much of a natural setting as possible within the San Dieguito River/Santa Ysabel Creek watershed, stretches about 50 miles between the coastline at Del Mar and Volcan Mountain near Julian. It follows the perimeter of freshwater wetlands of upper Lake Hodges near a crossroads originally known as Bernardo. A diverse community of birds and other wildlife calls this home.

The trailhead is the same as for Bernardo Mountain (Hike 10). Your first stop, only 500 feet from the trailhead, is the Sikes Adobe Historic Farmhouse, a circa 1870s structure and one of the San Diego region's oldest adobe homes from the American era. Designated a California Point of Historic Interest and a City of San Diego Historic Site, Sikes Adobe was restored in 2004 but sadly burned in the October 2007 Witch Fire, leaving only adobe walls standing. Rising like a phoenix following a second rebuilding, Sikes Adobe reopened in 2010. Administered by the San Dieguito River Park Joint Powers Authority and staffed with volunteer docents, the farmhouse and grounds are open to visitors for tours on Sundays, 10:30 a.m.–3:30 p.m., or by appointment. A small donation is recommended. If you can time your hike when the house is open, consider devoting 30 minutes or so to the interior tour to learn about Zenas Sikes's family and their pioneering farming life here in the Bernardo community in the 1870s and early 1880s.

Beyond the Sikes's grounds, Mule Hill Trail leads to a boulder-covered hill associated with the 1846 Battle of San Pasqual. Fought between U.S. Army troops under General Stephen Kearny and Californios under Captain Andrés Pico, this armed engagement was an effort to force back imposed US military rule at a time when California belonged to Mexico. A short but deadly skirmish took place 5 miles east of here. Famed scout Kit Carson was a participant in the battle and subsequent retreat to Mule Hill, so named because the Americans were forced to eat some of their mules while surrounded and under siege. An accounting of this event is presented on interpretive panels alongside the trail (and at San Pasqual Battlefield State Historic Park near the battle site, just east of the San Diego Zoo Safari Park).

THE ROUTE

Start from Sunset Drive and head east, away from I-15, beginning from a signed trailhead, and follow a wide dirt path leading in only 500 feet to the fenced Sikes Adobe grounds. A gate and kiosk will be on your left. If the adobe is open, the gate will be too. After passing the gate, the trail dips slightly to cross an intermittent stream, then circles around the perimeter of a golf driving range. At 0.45 mile, the trail comes to and parallels Via

Rancho Parkway where it transitions to Bear Valley Parkway. A shopping center is directly across the street to the north. After another 0.1 mile, the trail turns sharply right (south) and quickly leaves traffic noise behind as you enter a world rich with birdsong, the hum of bees, or perhaps the cries of a red-tailed hawk soaring above.

Just before the 0.75-mile point, you encounter the first interpretive plaque in a series describing phases of the battle and retreat to Mule Hill. Continue south with Mule Hill on your left. Just past the hill, also on the left, is a low wall made of river rock and three more plaques illustrating the 1846 standoff on Mule Hill. Another rock wall with four plaques provides an overview of the now-vanished town of Bernardo (1872–1917) and brief histories of earlier local features, including Rancho San Bernardo (1789–1872) and the San Diego to Yuma Road (1820–1870).

The trail now bends left (east) and ascends a low rise where it becomes the San Pasqual Valley Trail, a popular route for mountain biking and horseback riding. Your turnaround, 1.4 miles from the trailhead, is at this high point overlooking agricultural fields and a fine view back toward Mule Hill.

When you're ready to go, return the way you came.

TO THE TRAILHEAD
GPS Coordinates: N33º 3.993'   W117º 4.067'

Exit I-15 at Via Rancho Parkway (Exit 27) in south Escondido. Go east one long block to Sunset Drive. Turn right and drive 0.2 mile to the San Dieguito River Park trailhead and parking area.

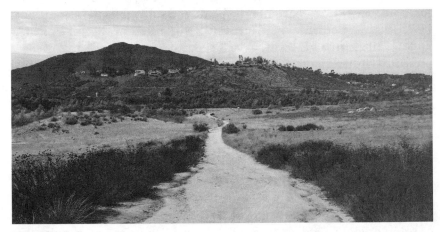

Mule Hill Trail

12 Jack Creek Meadow

Trailhead Location: North Escondido

Trail Use: Hiking, mountain biking, running, dog walking

Distance & Configuration: 5.6-mile balloon

Elevation Range: 1,180'–1,500'

Facilities: Water, restrooms, picnic grounds at Daley Ranch house, as well as in the Dixon Lake Recreation Area, near the trailhead

Highlights: Serene scenery, ranging from grassy meadow to oak woodland, nearly all of it in its natural state

DESCRIPTION

Daley Ranch preserve, a former working ranch that passed into public ownership in the 1990s, occupies the only large undeveloped acreage in the city of Escondido. Here, we spotlight the best introductory hike Daley Ranch offers, taking you to a remote elevated valley completely removed from the sights and sounds of civilization.

The hike or bike ride to Jack Creek Meadow is outstanding when taken during the cooler months, and it's tolerably comfortable on most summer days, assuming you travel in the early morning or late afternoon. If you live or work in inland North County, consider this route for a bit of quick and intense exercise: a speed walk of perhaps 90 minutes, a 60-minute jog, or a 40-minute mountain bike ride. The ranch property is open dawn to dusk.

THE ROUTE

At the Daley Ranch parking lot and staging area, step around the impressive Daley Ranch gate and walk uphill, rather steeply, on the paved access road ahead. Just beyond the gate, on the right side of the trail, an illustrated pocket guide to native plants published by Friends of Daley Ranch is available from a self-service box for a suggested donation of $2. Carry one along as an aid to identifying the signature plants found here in the three native habitats: oak woodlands, coastal sage scrub, and chaparral.

This service road, named Ranch House Trail, reaches a summit at 0.4 mile and then starts descending into live-oak woods. On the right, you get a glimpse of the largest of several old stock ponds on the ranch, its

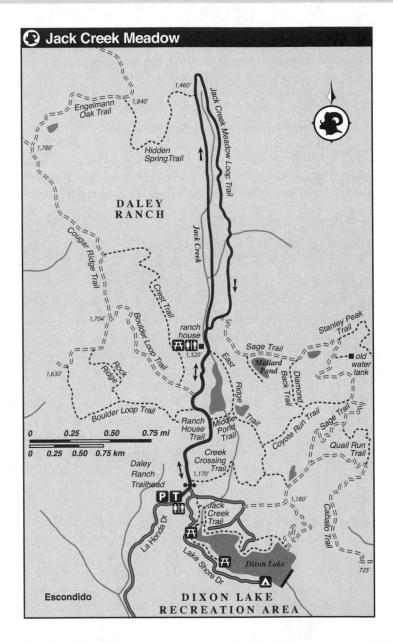

Jack Creek Meadow

shoreline guarded by tall cattails. Accessible from Middle Pond Trail and Sage/Mallard Trails (Mallard Pond), these ponds are great places for birding, especially after they have been refreshed with runoff from winter rains.

After 1.2 miles, pavement on Ranch House Trail ends at the quaint redwood Daley Ranch house. Descendants of Robert Daley, who settled in this valley in 1869, erected the house in 1928. It is generally closed to public visitation, but ranger-led tours are given the second Sunday of every month, 11 a.m.–2 p.m. Restrooms and water are available across the road from the ranch house. Continue north another 200 yards past two picnic areas, a barn, and various vintage outbuildings to the beginning of the dirt-road route signed as JACK CREEK MEADOW.

The elongated loop you follow—Jack Creek Meadow Loop Trail— takes you around the margins of a linear meadow, so narrow and so straight that it suggests some underlying, probably ancient, fault structure. The meadow, lined with a dark-green row of coast live oaks and backed up by steep slopes shaggy with mature chaparral, looks impressive when seen in early morning or late afternoon light. Close at hand you pass several gnarled specimens of Engelmann oak, with gray-green leaves and light-colored bark. You are likely to encounter tracks left by mule deer, coyotes, and raccoons and may even see one or more of these Daley Ranch residents, especially on weekdays when there are fewer visitors to interrupt their daily routines. Red-tailed hawks soaring or hunting along the perimeter ridges are a common sight. The meadow grasses are almost entirely nonnative, typically of an emerald-green color for about three months in the winter and bleached yellow-brown after one or two months of springtime sun and prolonged drought.

After completing the inspirational loop around the meadow, return to your car the way you came.

TO THE TRAILHEAD

GPS Coordinates: N33° 10.008'   W117° 3.119'

Exit I-15 at El Norte Parkway (Exit 33) in north Escondido. Drive 3.1 miles east and make a left turn (north) on La Honda Drive. Drive 1.3 miles uphill to the end of the road, where you will find the large parking lot and staging area for Daley Ranch on the left, just short of the Dixon Lake entrance. Overflow parking and restrooms are also available at Dixon Lake with free entry Monday–Thursday and a $5-per-vehicle charge on weekends.

13 San Pasqual Trails South

Trailhead Location: Between Escondido and Ramona in north-central San Diego County

Trail Use: Hiking, running, dog walking

Distance & Configuration: 6.4-mile out-and-back (including two spurs)

Elevation Range: 680' at the start to 1,755' at the highest point

Facilities: None near the trailhead; water and restrooms at San Pasqual Battlefield State Historic Park (if open), 4 miles west

Highlights: Spacious views of mountains, valleys, and the distant Pacific coastline

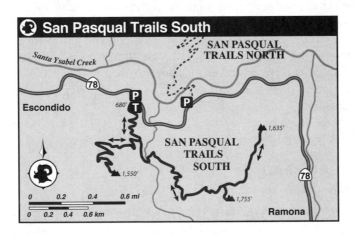

DESCRIPTION

The San Dieguito River Park's San Pasqual (also known as Clevenger Canyon) trail system lies within San Diego County's arid interior, east of Escondido. These trails expose you to steep, boulder-frosted hillsides, clothed in a tough mixture of vegetation that is recovering from the 2007 Guejito Fire. You'll see fast-growing sage scrub plants and slower-growing chaparral. Because of the high summer temperatures, it's best to hike in cool months. Here and there, you'll benefit from the shade of coast live oaks—hardy survivors that have seen many wildfires over a span of decades or longer.

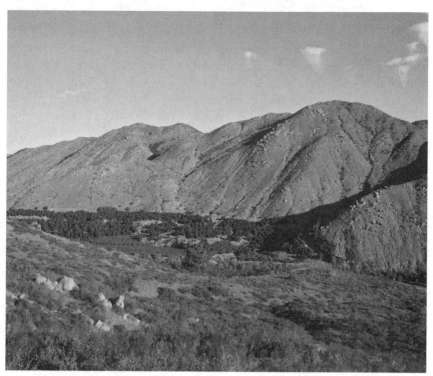

Looking north across San Pasqual Valley

The trail system consists of two networks, north and south of CA 78, but here we'll focus on the south trail system, which has been better maintained since the fire.

THE ROUTE

The complete reconnaissance of the southside trails involves a 6.4-mile round-trip. While the elevation ranges 680–1,755 feet, you will experience a *cumulative* elevation gain of 1,800 feet and loss of 1,800 feet. It's worth it: if you go on an unusually clear day, the coast-to-mountain views on the high points reached via these trails can be truly stunning.

Start your walk from the trailhead by zigzagging uphill 0.5 mile to the first marked trail junction. Choose the right branch (west) for a relatively easy climb to a 1,550-foot knoll. From this vantage point, you can spot the blue or silvery (depending on the time of day) ocean surface on clear winter days. An end-of-trail sign demarks your turnaround. Please don't continue farther to avoid impacting fragile habitat beyond this point.

Return the same way, and when you are back at the trail intersection, head up the more challenging east branch. You begin with a short passage through a spooky ravine, replete with a tangle of live-oak limbs, wild cucumber and poison oak vines, and a mantle of mosses. You cross two small wood plank bridges while passing through this section. On the far side, you tackle switchback segments of trail leading toward a prominent, monolithic boulder on a high ridge to the east. After passing within a few yards of the boulder, a side trail on the right leads to a 1,755-foot viewpoint—good for another view to the west. Return to the main east branch trail and continue toward a 1,635-foot bump on a ridge 0.5 mile northeast. Just right of the trail, at 0.2 mile beyond the 1,755-foot high point, you pass by a real novelty—two steel rocking chairs anchored to the top of a large boulder. A small use trail to the right (east) leads to the back of the boulder and wooden steps leading to the top. There's not much room up here except for the chairs, so watch your footing if you elect to pause here for an unforgettable experience.

From the chairs, it is a short 0.5-mile amble to the northeast overlook. That's where, on a clear day, you get a stupendous view of upper San Pasqual Valley, a slice of ocean horizon in the west, and the distant blue-tinted mountains in the east. Almost straight down 1,000 feet, you can spy cars, which appear toylike as they make their way along the sinuous asphalt ribbon of CA 78. Return to the trailhead along the main trail, bypassing your earlier side trips.

TO THE TRAILHEAD
GPS Coordinates: N33° 5.097'   W116° 55.328'

If coming from the south, take the I-15 exit at Via Rancho Parkway (Exit 27) south of Escondido. Turn right (east), and go 3.3 miles on Bear Valley Parkway. Turn right on CA 78, and go 8.6 miles.

If coming from the north, exit I-15 at CA 78 (Exit 32) and follow it east through several turns in Escondido toward the San Diego Zoo Safari Park. The San Pasqual South trailhead is located 5.5 miles east of the Safari Park entrance, on the right (south) side of CA 78.

14 Barnett Ranch Preserve

Trailhead Location: South of Ramona, in north-central San Diego County

Trail Use: Hiking, horseback riding, dog walking, mountain biking, running

Distance & Configuration: 5-mile out-and-back (including two spurs) or 4.3-mile loop

Elevation Range: 1,420'–1,520'

Facilities: A couple of picnic tables along the route; all other services in Ramona, 3 miles north

Highlights: Rolling grasslands reminiscent of Montana's Big Sky Country

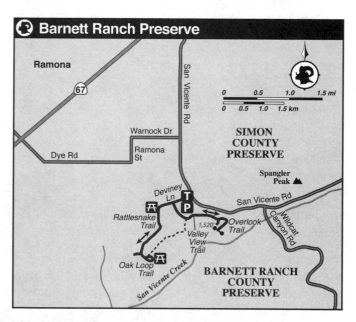

DESCRIPTION

Barnett Ranch County Preserve, operated by the county of San Diego, is one of several former cattle ranches converted in recent years to parkland throughout San Diego's suburban and rural areas. An ongoing project called the Multiple Species Conservation Program aims to protect key parcels such as this one for the benefit of indigenous flora and fauna, as well as for human visitors.

Barnett Ranch County Preserve spreads across about 728 acres of gently rolling grasslands and sage- and chaparral-covered slopes. The preserve offers multiuse trails (former unpaved ranch roads) that take you to nearly every corner of the property.

THE ROUTE

From the Barnett Ranch staging area, this outing includes two out-and-back multiuse routes: the Rattlesnake Trail and the Valley View Trail. The Rattlesnake Trail is terrific, once you get beyond the initial 0.5-mile dirt path alongside a rural driveway. You will curve into a sensuously rounded vale, cross a freshwater marsh with verdant grasses and swaying cattails (and a nearby bench), and climb a bit more to reach the Oak Loop Trail, a short 0.2-mile circuit featuring a picnic table set beneath a giant coast live oak, a hardy survivor of the 2003 Cedar Fire.

In the spring—March or April following a wet winter—the landscape looks as green as Ireland, and wildflowers pop up everywhere. This is also

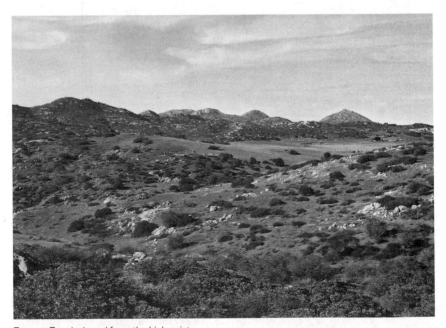

Barnett Ranch viewed from the high point

a prime area for observing migrating ferruginous hawks, North America's largest buteo, snowbirding in the Ramona Valley during winter months. On a summer visit, you'll likely spot ravens, red-tailed hawks, and perhaps a majestic golden eagle soaring overhead. Under the warm sun, minivortexes of heated air might carve raspy-sounding grooves through the dry grasses, like ghosts dancing.

Reverse your route and return to paved Deviney Lane and walk another 0.2 mile to a signed junction for Valley View Trail. Turn right (south) and follow the dirt road to a fork at a low wooden fence at 0.25 mile. The right fork, an informal use trail, connects back to Oak Loop and Rattlesnake Trails. For our hike take the left fork to stay on Valley View Trail. After passing over 0.5 mile of gently rolling grassland terrain graced with attractively shaped and spaced coast live oaks, you will come to the Overlook Trail. Turn right (south) and walk about 100 yards to reach the first overlook and perhaps the best perspective for seeing the full extent of the preserve. Return to the main trail, turn right (east), and continue slightly downhill 0.3 mile to the second viewpoint and a property gate marking the end of this trail. Pause here for a few minutes to take in a panorama looking out over chaparral-covered slopes of San Vicente Creek's valley dotted with various dwellings and ranching infrastructure. Return the way you came, and take a right at the intersection with Deviney Lane to arrive back at the trailhead.

For a slightly shorter option, consider taking advantage of the unofficial connector between Oak Loop Trail and Valley View Trail. According to county officials, it is acceptable to use this shortcut even though it is not signed nor does it show up on the park map. It can be hiked in either direction for a clockwise or counterclockwise loop depending on which spur you prefer to do first. The distance with the shortcut is 4.3 miles, including the out-and-back to Valley View.

TO THE TRAILHEAD
GPS Coordinates: N33° 0.035'   W116° 51.881'

From the junction of CA 67 and CA 78 in the center of Ramona, turn south on 10th Street. Within four blocks, 10th Street becomes San Vicente Road. Continue a total of 3 miles to Deviney Lane on the right (west) side of San Vicente Road. The well-marked trailhead and equestrian staging area for Barnett Ranch lies here. For some travelers, a shortcut to San Vicente Road from CA 67 via Dye Road, Ramona Street, and Warnock Drive might save time.

15 Blue Sky Ecological Reserve

Trailhead Location: Northern Poway

Trail Use: Hiking, dog walking, running, horseback riding

Distance & Configuration: 4.8-mile out-and-back

Elevation Range: 703' at the start to 1,350' at Lake Ramona Dam

Facilities: Portable toilet at the trailhead and 1 mile in

Highlights: Dense riparian and oak woodlands, as well as scenic views from Lake Ramona Dam

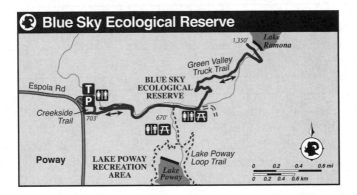

DESCRIPTION

The 700-acre Blue Sky Ecological Reserve near Poway protects one of the finest examples of riparian (streamside) vegetation in Southern California. As one of the most popular of the California Department of Fish and Wildlife reserves in the state, much attention here is focused on nature education, as well as habitat preservation. Motorized vehicles and mountain bikes are banned, so you'll be assured of peace and quiet, and more frequent wildlife sightings, as you stroll along. For dog owners looking for a fun group activity, organized dog walks start from the Blue Sky parking lot at 8 a.m. on the first Sunday of the month, October–June.

After a wet winter, usually by March, the reserve landscape turns an almost unbelievably bright shade of green. Mosses, ferns, annual grasses, and fresh new shrub growth coat everything, even the rocks. Wildflowers appear in great numbers by about April and start to fade by June, after the grasses have bleached to a straw-yellow color. More than 100 kinds of wildflowers have been identified here in a single year.

THE ROUTE

From the trailhead, follow the unpaved Green Valley Truck Trail along the south bank of a creek. Traffic noise disappears, and frogs entertain you with their guttural serenades. Live oaks spread their limbs overhead, casting pools of shade, while willows, sycamores, and lush thickets of poison oak cluster along the creek itself. Small illustrated signs along the route help with identification of a variety of native plants found along this wooded section of trail.

About 0.3 mile out, a fork on the left (north) leads to the Creekside Trail, heading toward the creek itself and paralleling the main trail for 0.5 mile, including a small loop (Oak Grove Trail) at the west end. Along this alternate path you can spot tadpoles, frogs, and perhaps other amphibious creatures. At the east end, a narrower path takes you back to the truck trail. Consider this option for either the outbound or return portions of your hike. One caution, though: The sheer volume of poison oak growth off the main truck trail cannot be overemphasized; learn to recognize the plant's leaves-of-three pattern, and keep your pets well away!

Note: At 0.9 mile, a trail branching right (south) heads uphill to join the trail system of the Lake Poway Recreation Area (Hike 16, page 61). Just beyond this junction, also on the right, is a picnic area occasionally used as an outdoor classroom in conjunction with the reserve's amphitheater located just east of the parking lot. About 0.2 mile farther on the main road, where you will see power lines overhead, there's a major split. The left branch (Green Valley Truck Trail) fords the creek and starts climbing, as do you, a dry south-facing slope toward the Lake Ramona Dam. In the next 1.3 miles of steady ascent, you'll gain about 700 feet of elevation and enjoy an ever-expanding view of inland San Diego County's mix of suburban development and open space. If it's a hot summer day, you might want to forego for the time being that last 1.3 miles, which offer little or no shade.

Once you reach the dam and reservoir, you can turn around and return on the same route or walk across the dam, adding about 0.8 mile round-trip and providing fine views in both directions. Fortunately the hike back is downhill all the way.

Within 0.1 mile of the trailhead and 0.1 mile after the last junction for Creekside Trail, another trail to the right (north) has a small sign

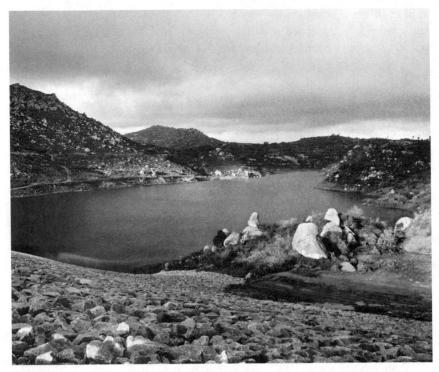

Lake Ramona

identifying it as the Torretto Outlook Trail. As an option, take this loop path up to a modest overlook to the east, then pass the outdoor amphitheater to reach the parking lot and trailhead in 0.25 mile.

TO THE TRAILHEAD

GPS Coordinates: N33° 0.961'   W117° 1.422'

Exit I-15 at Rancho Bernardo Road (Exit 24) and go east. Rancho Bernardo Road becomes Espola Road as you enter Poway city limits. Espola curves south after about 3 miles. The Blue Sky Ecological Reserve entrance is on the left, just after the curve, 3.4 miles from I-15. The gated parking lot is open November–May, daily, sunrise–sunset, and June–October, daily, 6:30 a.m.–sunset.

16 Lake Poway Loop

Trailhead Location: Eastern Poway

Trail Use: Hiking, dog walking, running, mountain biking, horseback riding

Distance & Configuration: 2.7-mile loop

Elevation Range: 760'–1,115'

Facilities: Water, restrooms, and picnic areas at the start with portable restrooms available along the route on east and south sides of the lake

Highlights: Heart-pumping exercise while circumnavigating a scenic reservoir

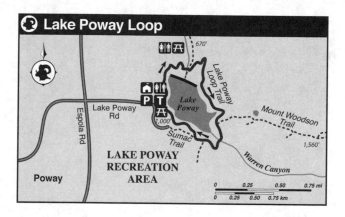

DESCRIPTION

Like most of San Diego County's water reservoirs, Lake Poway stores water imported through aqueducts from the Colorado River and from Northern California. Fortunately, the city of Poway included a strong recreational element in the plan for this reservoir, which resulted in a wealth of opportunities for the lake and its surroundings: picnicking, hiking, boating, fishing, and group camping. Nonresidents pay a $10-per-vehicle entry fee on weekends and holidays, but access is free to everyone Monday–Thursday.

The looping trail around Lake Poway provides an excellent exercise opportunity for runners and walkers, with a good mixture of flats, gentle hills, and a few fairly steep switchbacks. On the trail, you'll pass through four distinct plant communities: sage scrub, chaparral, oak woodland, and riparian woodland.

THE ROUTE
Find the Lake Poway Loop Trail just beyond the lake entrance, to the left of the park office and concession building. The trail follows the west shoreline to as far as the rock-fill Harry W. Frame Dam, descends to a creek crossing, and soon reaches a dirt maintenance road. Turn left (north) and stay with that road for about 100 yards, where you will see

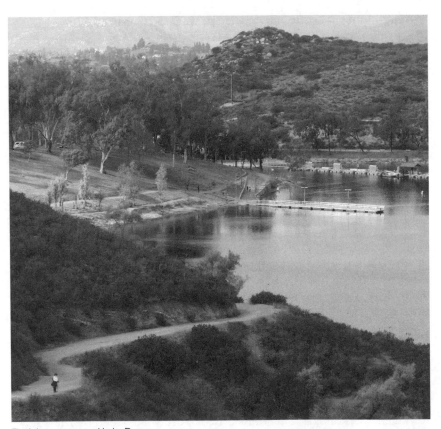
Final descent toward Lake Poway

the Lake Poway Loop Trail continuing on the right. At that juncture, if you want, you can make a short side trip north for 0.1 mile down to a picnic area (formerly a wilderness campground) in the Blue Sky Ecological Preserve, a walk-in or ride-in site for hikers and equestrians. Tables and flush toilets are available here.

Follow the trail as it resumes climbing generally east, away from the dirt road. By way of a lengthy zigzag and a couple of smaller wiggles in the trail, you gain a slope above the east buttress of the dam. Press on, traversing easily around the east shoreline, and note the junction of the Mount Woodson Trail on the left, which provides eastern access to the summit and ever-popular Potato Chip Rock. Keep going straight, circling around the south arm of the lake and past an overlook with benches, a great spot to pause and take in one of the best views of Lake Poway. Descend from the overlook along the main trail, skipping three junctions to the left associated with the Sumac Trail, to arrive at the lawn area and boat dock just shy of where you started the loop hike.

TO THE TRAILHEAD
GPS Coordinates: N33° 0.409'   W117° 0.807'

About 25 miles north of central San Diego, exit I-15 at Rancho Bernardo Road (Exit 24) in Rancho Bernardo; head east. Rancho Bernardo Road becomes Espola Road as you enter Poway's city limits. Espola starts to curve south after about 3 miles. Drive a total of 4 miles from I-15 to reach Lake Poway Road. Turn left (east) there, and drive 0.5 mile to the Lake Poway Recreation Area, where plenty of parking space is available near the park office and trailhead.

17 Iron Mountain

Trailhead Location: East of Poway in north-central San Diego County

Trail Use: Hiking, running, dog walking, mountain biking, horseback riding

Distance & Configuration: 5.8-mile out-and-back

Elevation Range: 1,611' at the start to 2,696' at the summit

Facilities: Restrooms and drinking water at the trailhead parking area

Highlights: A leisurely, seldom-steep ascent; ocean-to-mountain vistas as you approach the summit

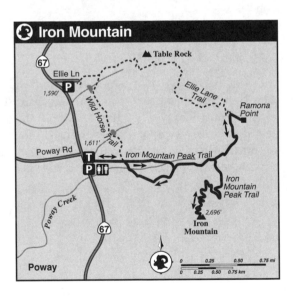

DESCRIPTION

Poway's Iron Mountain thrusts its conical, chaparral-clad summit nearly 2,700 feet above sea level, a height that is frequently well above the low-lying coastal haze. On many a crystalline winter day, the summit offers a sweeping, 360-degree panorama from glistening ocean to blue mountains and back to the ocean again. The main trail to the summit, 2.9 miles one way, is smoothly graded and hardly falters in its steady elevation gain. All kinds of self-propelled travelers use this popular trail, though mountain bikers and equestrians aren't seen much. On pleasant weekends, hundreds of hikers converge on this trail for their morning exercise.

THE ROUTE

From the trailhead parking lot, pass beneath the wood and wrought iron signed arch that frames the peak. Angle right a short distance to meet the original trailhead from the days before the parking lot and restroom structure were constructed. Head east on the wide and almost level Iron Mountain Peak Trail, flanked initially on both sides by rows of planted trees. Ignore the trail branching left (north), the Wild Horse Trail, and the one to the right (south) that offers an optional return path. Continue on the main trail to a spot about 1 mile into the hike, where the trail narrows and briefly dips to cross the bottom of a ravine that may feature a small seasonal creek following winter rains. On the far side of the ravine, you climb in earnest for a while, negotiating the steepest grade you'll encounter along the whole route.

At 1.5 miles you reach a saddle where you can turn left or right. Stay right (south) and commence a generally leisurely ascent through the low-growing coastal sage scrub and chaparral. Prior to the mid-1990s, the chaparral grew thick and tall here, sometimes high enough to form a tunnel overhead. Now, after two major wildfires, Iron Mountain's vegetation struggles to reach a climax phase, which takes at least 25–30 years of slow and steady growth.

After a definitive turn to the west, the ascent on the trail becomes steeper again, and final switchbacks take you back and forth across the ever-narrowing summit cone of Iron Mountain. On the boulders at the top, you will see a massive, pier-mounted telescope (no coins required) thoughtfully placed so anyone can scan the near and far horizons. You may also see a visitor register—a notebook stuffed with hundreds of written comments. Return to the main trail via the same route.

If you are still aching to get in more of a workout, consider the following bonus option. At the saddle junction, turn right. It is only 0.75 mile to Ramona Point, just south of impressive cliffs and a view straight down Ramona's Main Street (CA 67). When you are ready to return, head south back to the saddle junction. After descending from the saddle for 0.5 mile and at the last switchback before crossing the ravine, an alternate trail heads to your left. It is about the same distance as the main trail and comes out at the Wild Horse Trail. This path is less rocky or exposed than the way you came up and passes through a corridor of more mature, close-to-the-trail vegetation, somewhat reminiscent of pre-wildfire conditions on Iron Mountain.

TO THE TRAILHEAD

GPS Coordinates: N32° 58.694'   W116° 58.353'

On I-15, about 15 miles north of central San Diego, exit at Scripps Poway Parkway (Exit 17). Follow Scripps Poway Parkway east 9 miles to its end at CA 67. Turn left on CA 67 and drive 2 miles north to the traffic light at Poway Road. The 100-space Iron Mountain staging area and trailhead lie on the right. On weekends, this parking lot may fill up; overflow parking is allowed along the CA 67 shoulder.

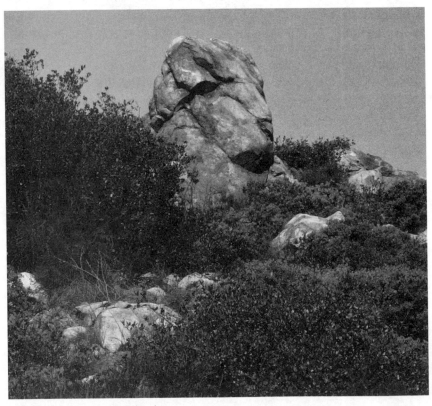

A rock in the shape of a dog's head

18 Woodson Mountain

Trailhead Location: Between Poway and Ramona, in north-central San Diego County

Trail Use: Hiking, dog walking, running, biking, night hiking

Distance & Configuration: 4-mile out-and-back

Elevation Change: 1,680' at the start to 2,894' at the summit

Facilities: No facilities nearby other than in Ramona or Poway, each several miles away

Highlights: Outsize boulders pepper the slopes of this wild-looking mountain. Topside views are some of the broadest in San Diego County.

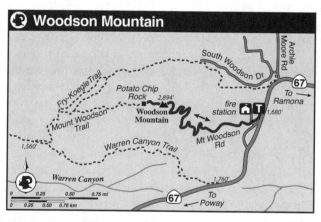

DESCRIPTION

Local American Indians called it Mountain of Moonlit Rocks in their language, an appropriate moniker for a landmark visible, even at night, from great distances. Later, settlers dubbed it Cobbleback Peak, a name utterly descriptive of its rugged, boulder-strewn slopes. But for more than a century, the peak has appeared on maps simply as Woodson Mountain, after Confederate doctor Marshall Clay Woodson, who homesteaded at its foot in 1875. Today, Woodson Mountain is a local landmark, renowned among rock climbers all over Southern California, as well as among local hikers, who are able to ascend the peak from a variety of directions.

The eastern approach described here uses a paved service road closed to motor traffic. Though very steep in places, the smooth-surfaced path lends itself well to after-dark hiking, provided you have a headlamp or flashlight. The route is also suitable for road and mountain biking, but that's practical only if your bike has extremely low gears and the brakes are in tip-top shape.

Summer days are typically too hot for climbing Woodson. Early morning or late afternoon sometimes works spectacularly, though. At those times, during much of the warmer half of the year, stratus clouds cover the coastal landscape up to an elevation of 1,000–2,000 feet. Woodson's 2,894-foot summit often pokes above that dense blanket of cottony clouds, much to the pleasure of early-morning visitors. Incredible sunset views often reward late-afternoon or evening hikes, and that advantage is doubled whenever there's a full moon. With every full moon on a clear evening, you can witness a near-simultaneous sunset in the west and moonrise in the east.

THE ROUTE

A small sign marks the trailhead at the entrance to the fire station. From that starting point, follow a narrow path south through some oak trees alongside CA 67. Within only 0.1 mile, you arrive at the paved service road. Turn right and chug 1.7 miles up, up, and up to Woodson's antenna-topped summit, some 1,200 feet higher than your starting point. Everywhere you look, there are rounded boulders galore. The beige and light-gray rocks of Woodson Mountain and several of its neighboring peaks are what geologists call Woodson Mountain granodiorite. When exposed at the surface, they weather into huge spherical or ellipsoidal boulders with smooth surfaces. The largest of them have a tendency to cleave apart along remarkably flat planes, leaving gaps of several inches to several feet. Sometimes, half of a split boulder will roll away, leaving a vertical and almost seamless face behind. Near the top of the mountain, you'll feel absolutely dwarfed as you pass between boulders the size of large houses.

As you approach the summit, the incline moderates somewhat, and you can catch your breath. On the summit itself you'll have to move around a bit, dodging antenna installations, for views in every direction. To enjoy the optimum western view, walk about 0.2 mile farther west and downhill from the summit, along the narrow summit ridge. After passing several antenna towers, you'll reach a vantage point overlooking Poway and much of the North County, not to mention a vast sweep of the Pacific Ocean—if the atmosphere is clear enough. Very near that spot, don't miss the sight of an amazing cantilevered "potato chip" flake of rock, the result of exfoliation and weathering of a huge boulder. The coauthor suspects the current name—Potato Chip

Rock—can be attributed to one of Jerry's route descriptions dating back to the third edition of *Afoot & Afield: San Diego County,* published in 1998. His apt description has been retained here as it appeared then, as well as in the first edition of *50 Best Short Hikes: San Diego.* Following widely viewed YouTube videos and online postings, this feature now attracts hundreds of visitors every weekend. They make the trek up from either the west or east trailheads, and a line often forms early as hikers take turns to have photos taken while they pose on this seemingly death-defying precipice.

When it's time to leave, head back the same way you came. The traction on the paved road is excellent, but it's a real knee banger due to the steep slope.

TO THE TRAILHEAD
GPS Coordinates: N33° 0.499'   W116° 57.327'

The starting point is a marked trailhead just off the west shoulder of CA 67 near the entrance to a California Division of Forestry fire station at the eastern base of Woodson Mountain. From the intersection of Poway Road and CA 67 in Poway, travel north on CA 67 for 3 miles. The trailhead is on your left (west).

From the CA 67 and CA 78 intersection in Ramona, drive southwest for 6 miles. The trailhead is on your right (west). Park on the wide eastside shoulder or on the narrower westside shoulder of CA 67. Do not park on fire station property. Please use care when crossing ever-busy CA 67. As this is one of the most popular hikes in San Diego, finding parking right next to the trailhead can be a challenge, especially on weekends.

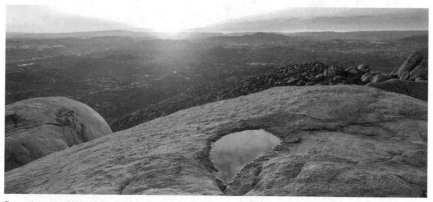

Summit area of Woodson Mountain

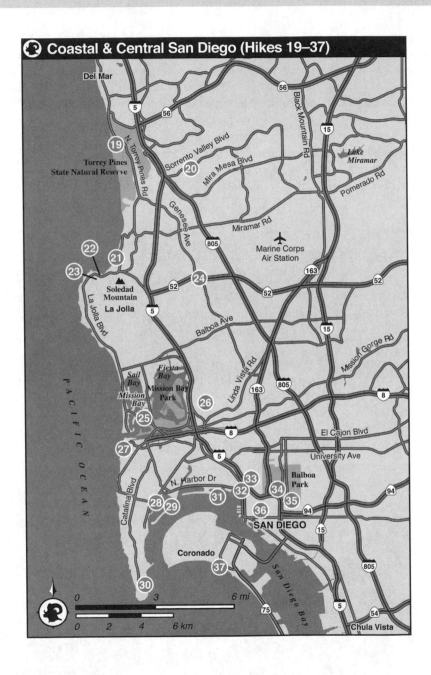

Coastal & Central San Diego (Hikes 19–37)

Del Mar

56

5

56

Black Mountain Rd

15

19

Sorrento Valley Blvd

20

Mira Mesa Blvd

Lake Miramar

N. Torrey Pines Rd

Torrey Pines State Natural Reserve

Genesee Ave

Pomerado Rd

Miramar Rd

805

Marine Corps Air Station

163

52

22

21

23

Soledad Mountain

La Jolla

52

24

52

52

15

La Jolla Blvd

5

Balboa Ave

Mission Gorge Rd

Sail Bay

Fiesta Bay

Linda Vista Rd

Mission Bay

Mission Bay Park

163

805

8

26

25

8

El Cajon Blvd

27

5

University Ave

Catalina Blvd

N. Harbor Dr

33

Balboa Park

28 29

31

32

34

94

36

35

94

30

SAN DIEGO

15

Coronado

San Diego Bay

37

805

0   3   6 mi

75

5

0   2   4   6 km

54

Chula Vista

COASTAL & CENTRAL SAN DIEGO

Urban San Diego's landscape differs from that of most other densely populated cities. Outside its compact downtown, the city is a vast collection of distinct neighborhoods, some hugging the coast and others spreading inland.

San Diego's predominant canyon, mesa, and river valley topography ensures that not every acre of the city could, or would, be built upon. This, of course, is great news for urban hikers.

In addition to dozens of canyonside open spaces, San Diego has a long tradition of setting aside large tracts of land for use as city parks. One outstanding example is 1,200-acre Balboa Park, established in 1868 but not developed extensively before the early 1900s. A more recent example is Mission Bay Park, with 27 miles of shoreline. The latter's creation involved the conversion of mudflats into a modern-day, water-oriented recreational space.

Aside from these hiking and walking venues, opportunities abound for walks that highlight architectural and historic features. For example, relatively few locals, let alone tourists, are aware of the charming and intriguing footbridges spanning urban canyons just north of downtown. Even the core of downtown San Diego can offer up worthwhile viewing that simply would be missed if experienced by any conveyance other than on foot.

Central San Diego's proximity to the ocean goes hand in hand with year-round mild weather conditions. Another plus for hiking on nearly all of the routes within this section is that access to drinking water is of little concern, thanks to the nearby availability of public facilities, along with restaurants and small cafés.

You may, no doubt, face parking challenges on several of the hikes included in this section. However, as appropriate, the profiles will give you tips on where to begin the walk near reasonable parking areas.

■ ◘ ■

19 Torrey Pines State Natural Reserve

Trailhead Location: Just south of Del Mar

Trail Use: Hiking, running

Distance & Configuration: 1–4 miles on looping and out-and-back trails

Elevation Range: Sea level to 350'

Facilities: Water and restrooms at the trailheads

Highlights: Magnificent ocean vistas, rare flora, and nearly perfect year-round climate

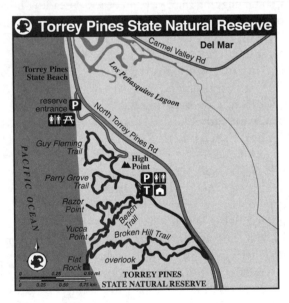

DESCRIPTION

The rare and beautiful Torrey pine trees atop the coastal bluffs south of Del Mar are as much a symbol of the Golden State as are the famed Monterey cypress trees native to California's central coast. Torrey pines grow naturally in only two places on Earth: in and around Torrey Pines State Natural Reserve and on Santa Rosa Island, off Santa Barbara.

Torrey Pines State Natural Reserve would be botanically noteworthy even without its pines. More than 330 species of plants have been identified there so far. Sage scrub, chaparral, and salt marsh plant communities are present in various parts of the reserve.

If you're interested in identifying plants and wildflowers typical of the coast and coastal strip, the reserve is simply the best single place to go in San Diego County. Excellent interpretive facilities at the reserve's visitor center make this an easy task. Besides the exhibits, you can browse through several notebooks full of captioned photographs of common and rare plants within the reserve. You can also visit the native plant gardens surrounding the visitor building and at the head of the Parry Grove Trail.

If you visit the reserve a number of times during February–June, you'll be able to follow the succession of flowering as the spring season progresses. Wildflower maps, updated monthly, are often available.

THE ROUTE

Assuming you start at the reserve's main trailhead, a stone's throw from the visitor center, you'll have your choice of a variety of short- to moderate-length hikes, none involving more than 350 feet of elevation loss and gain. If you elect to try all of the trails in a single go, expect to cover nearly 8 miles, including the connector routes.

For an overview of the entire area, you might first try the 100-yard-long trail to High Point, opposite the Parry Grove Trail, just north of the visitor center. You'll enjoy a panoramic view of the pine-clad uplands of the reserve, the ocean, and the flat, green Los Peñasquitos Lagoon just east.

Next, you might head south on an antique concrete segment of the original Coast Highway, just south of the visitor center, and pick up the Broken Hill Trail. The two east branches of this trail wind through dense chaparral just north of world-famous Torrey Pines Golf Course. Either will connect to a spur trail leading to Broken Hill Overlook. You'll be able to step out (carefully) onto a precipitous fin of sandstone and peer over to see what looks like desert badlands. A third (west) branch of the Broken Hill Trail winds down a slope festooned with wildflowers and joins the Beach Trail at a point just above where the latter drops sharply to the beach.

The popular Beach Trail originates at the visitor center trailhead and heads downward toward the beach, intersecting with side trails to Yucca Point and Razor Point along the way. From these side destinations, you can peer nearly straight down to the sandy beach and surf. If you follow Beach Trail all the way down to the beach itself, any further travel would likely be blocked by high water during the highest tides, especially in winter, when strong wave action tends to strip sand away from the beach. At times of lower tides, and more often in summer and fall, you could head north along the sand and reach the reserve's entrance, 1 mile north.

Back to the Parry Grove and Guy Fleming Trails, both north of the visitor center, you will wind among the most extensive groves of Torrey pines. Prolonged dry spells over the past 30 years or so—plus a resurgence of bark beetles—killed many of the large trees, especially those on the drier, south-facing slopes. Seedlings have been planted here and there in an effort to restore these groves to their former glory.

The Guy Fleming Trail, named for the reserve's first caretaker, is mostly flat, while the Parry Grove Trail starts with a steep descent on stone steps. In spring, the sunny slopes along the Guy Fleming Trail come alive with phantasmagoric wildflower displays. Fluttering in the sea breeze, the flowers put on quite a show as several vivid shades of color dynamically intermix with the more muted tones of earth, sea, and sky.

You can't picnic on any of the reserve's trails (no food is allowed), but after you do your hiking, you can use the tables or the beach near the entrance. As with all hiking, do take water along on the trails. Also bring binoculars: ravens, red-tailed hawks, and peregrine falcons are reliably seen, as are humans lazily soaring about on paragliders. The gliders launch from nearby Torrey Pines Gliderport. You might even catch sight of an osprey diving into the shallow nearshore waters to grab, then lift off with, an unlucky fish. Be mindful that the reserve closes at sunset and plan to return before the gate closes.

TO THE TRAILHEAD
GPS Coordinates: N32° 55.192'   W117° 15.180'

Exit I-5 at Carmel Valley Road (Exit 33 or 33B). Drive 1.5 miles west to the Coast Highway (signed as CAMINO DEL MAR to the north and NORTH TORREY PINES ROAD to the south). Go left and proceed 0.8 mile south to the Torrey Pines State Natural Reserve parking lot on the right (fee charged), or find a parking spot for free along the Coast Highway. You also may enter the reserve entrance, pay the fee, and drive about 1 mile farther to the visitor center and main trailhead at the top of the coastal bluffs.

20 Los Peñasquitos Canyon

Trailhead Location: East of Del Mar

Trail Use: Hiking, running, mountain biking, dog walking, horseback riding

Distance & Configuration: 5.5-mile out-and-back

Elevation Range: 60' at the start to 185'

Facilities: Portable restroom at the trailhead

Highlights: A cascading waterfall following winter rains

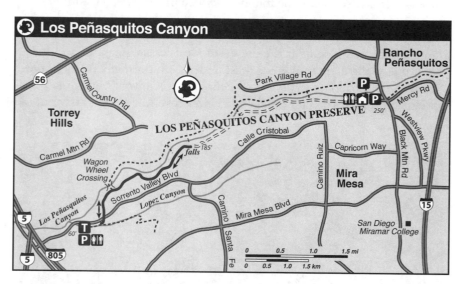

DESCRIPTION

Crickets sing and bullfrogs groan. A hawk alights upon a sycamore limb and then launches with outstretched wings to catch a puff of sea breeze moving up the canyon. Perhaps a white-tailed kite hovers facing into the wind, then drops quickly to the ground to snatch an unseen mouse or vole. A cottontail rabbit bounds across the trail and stops to take your measure with a sidelong stare. Los Peñasquitos Creek, rejuvenated by winter rains, slips silently through a sparkling pool and darts noisily down multiple paths in the constriction known as the falls.

Despite miles of suburban development surrounding it, Los Peñasquitos Canyon Preserve still retains its gentle, unselfconscious beauty. The preserve's 4,000 acres of San Diego city- and county-owned open space stretch
for almost 7 miles between the I-5/I-805 merge and I-15, encompassing
much of Los Peñasquitos Creek and one of its tributaries, Lopez Canyon.
Aside from historic dwellings and ruins dating back to the mid-1800s, the
preserve hosts a trail system popular with every sort of self-propelled traveler.

The falls lie nearly at the midpoint of a 6-mile-long, unspoiled segment
of Los Peñasquitos Canyon; they are equally accessible from the east or the
west via a wide pathway—the unpaved access road that ran the length of
the canyon in its cattle-ranch days.

Here, we profile the west approach to the falls, which offers spacious
views of the canyon bottom and hillsides, plus some of the finest springtime wildflower scenery to be found anywhere in San Diego County.

THE ROUTE

From your starting point at the preserve's westside staging area and trailhead, follow the main trail going west underneath Sorrento Valley Boulevard and up broad and shallow Los Peñasquitos Canyon. Sometimes fine
springtime displays of lupine and owl's clover cover the steep, grassy slopes

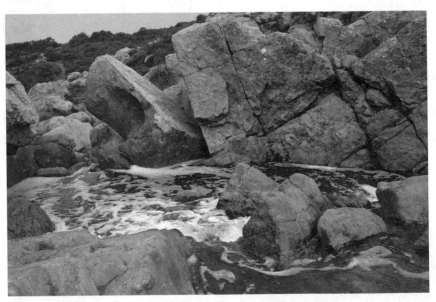

Main pool above waterfall

on the right. Wild radish, a plant introduced from Europe, often paints the lower slopes with shades of blue, white, and purple.

At about 0.7 mile, the trail comes close to the creek, and there's a creek crossing on the left leading to a singletrack trail on the far side (Wagon Wheel Crossing). This is only the first of several minor side trails in the next several miles that link to pathways on the far bank. Your way, however, sticks to the main trail, which remains on the right (south) bank.

The main trail eventually climbs a small hill and then descends to more grassland, dotted with small trees and shrubs such as elderberry, live oak, laurel sumac, toyon, and gooseberry. Large sycamores and cottonwoods flank the creek to your left.

At about 2.5 miles into the hike, the trail starts curving up a chaparral-covered slope. Near the top, there's a wide spot with racks for securing bikes and a foot trail descending north to the falls area, where the Los Peñasquitos stream has carved a narrow constriction into the bedrock. Watch your footing here as the rock can be quite slippery.

When the flow of water is sufficient, typically January–May, water exuberantly cascades through here. Polished rock 10 feet up on either side testifies to its maximum depth in flood stage. The greenish-gray outcrops responsible for the cascading path of the water are a type of erosion-resistant metavolcanic rock (sediments formed from volcanic rock, then hardened by heat and pressure) dating to the late Jurassic period, over 140 million years ago, when this region was offshore and far to the south in Mexico. When the weather is warm, be vigilant in the area around the falls because rattlesnakes may be out and about.

When it's time to return, use the same route you traveled to get here.

TO THE TRAILHEAD
GPS Coordinates: N32° 54.391'   W117° 12.365'

Exit I-805 at Mira Mesa Boulevard/Sorrento Valley Road (Exit 27 or 27B). Take either I-805 frontage road (Sorrento Valley Road on the west side; Vista Sorrento Parkway on the east side) 1 mile north to Sorrento Valley Boulevard. Turn right and continue 1.1 miles east to a marked trailhead and staging area for Los Peñasquitos Canyon Preserve, on the right (south). The parking area is open sunrise–sunset.

21 La Jolla Shores

Trailhead Location: La Jolla

Trail Use: Hiking, running

Distance & Configuration: 2-mile to 3-mile out-and-back

Elevation Range: Sea level all the way

Facilities: Water and restrooms at Kellogg Park

Highlights: One of California's finest stretches of coastline, with a sandy beach, dramatic sea bluffs, and tidepools all within a short stretch

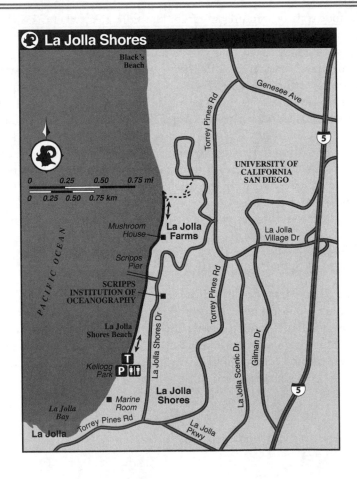

DESCRIPTION

For beachcombing, tidepool exploration, and all-over suntanning, La Jolla Shores Beach and the coastal stretch north of it can't be beat. It's important to note, though, that some of the better attributes of this environment aren't available at higher tides—typically 3 feet or more. In fact, the highest tides of up to 7 feet will limit your walk along the beach to only 0.5 mile each way, assuming you don't want to be swamped by waves. Extreme low tides (expressed on tide tables as 0 feet to −2 feet), on the other hand, are perfect for viewing marine life amid the rocky outcrops that lie at the lowest levels of the intertidal zone.

The timing of extreme low tides depends on the time of year. October–March, the extreme lows (which coincide with new and full moons) tend to occur during afternoon hours. April–September, similarly low tides are confined to the predawn hours—not great for those who value their sleep.

THE ROUTE

You'll begin walking on the beach adjacent to the grassy area known as Kellogg Park. Walk north on the sand, passing under the cliff-hugging buildings of Scripps Institution of Oceanography. The initial stretch of sand is gently shelving, extremely wide, and a pleasure to enjoy with bare feet during low-tide episodes. On the wet sand nearest the waves, you might catch shimmery reflections of Scripps Pier and looming Torrey Pines bluffs beyond.

You pass under Scripps Pier after about 0.5 mile. Just ahead, the cliffs on the right get taller and pinch in toward the water. You're on sandstone rocks and boulders now, wet and slippery near the waves and smooth and dry higher up, so put your shoes back on. The rocky tidepool area exposed during low tide is visibly wriggling with plant and animal life. The sea vegetation tends to move to and fro with the waves at the water's edge, while the sea creatures—including tiny fish, sea stars, shore and hermit crabs, and even octopuses—flit about at variable rates of speed. Please note that all species are protected here, and no collecting is allowed. It is always best to look but don't pick up.

Near the end of the tidepools, notice the narrow finger, or *dike* in geologic parlance, of grayish volcanic rock stretching diagonally out to sea, toward the southwest. This is the only significant exposure of volcanic rock along San Diego County's coastline. It dates from some 14 million years ago, in the Miocene epoch, when a pulse of magma pushed its way up nearly to Earth's surface.

Right after you pass the dike, the sandy beach resumes, flanked by tall cliffs on the right, crashing surf on the left, and an incredible circular structure nestled against the base of these bluffs and accessed by a nearly vertical 300-foot tramway. Known locally as the Mushroom House, it was built in 1969 as a guesthouse for the property above and features panoramic views from Torrey Pines to La Jolla. What gorgeous sunsets must have been seen from here over the years! You might want to slip off your shoes again and enjoy the feel of the fine, clean sand underfoot.

By that point, or not far ahead, you may notice that some beachgoers have doffed more than just shoes. You're now on Black's Beach, San Diego's ever-popular nude bathing and sunbathing spot. The warmer the weather, the more skin is exposed here. So, for whatever reasons you want, you can either turn back here, for this 2-mile round-trip walk, or continue north for literally miles ahead. Another good turnaround option is at a pedestrian ramp 0.5 mile ahead on the right that provides access to Black's Beach for University of California San Diego students and neighbors via a gated road and a long, steep 0.5-mile descent of a side canyon starting from La Jolla Farms Road. If you press on forward along the beach, do so *only if you have checked the tide tables for that day*. It is imperative that you remain mindful of any incoming higher tide that might swamp your return route.

TO THE TRAILHEAD
GPS Coordinates: N32° 51.471'   W117° 15.406'

From northbound I-5 (Exit 26A) or westbound CA 52 (Exit 1A), take La Jolla Parkway 2 miles west toward La Jolla. La Jolla Parkway merges into Torrey Pines Road. Immediately after, turn right on La Jolla Shores Drive at the fourth traffic light west of I-5, an intersection with a gas station on your right (north). Go five or six blocks north and turn left on narrow residential streets leading west to Kellogg Park, where a large parking lot lies between two spacious grassy areas. This lot can fill quickly, especially on weekends and during summer months, so plan on arriving early. Street parking is available but may involve a walk of several blocks to reach the beach. Even during the busiest periods, spaces can be found on side streets east of La Jolla Shores Drive.

22 Coast Walk

Trailhead Location: La Jolla

Trail Use: Hiking, dog walking, running

Distance & Configuration: 1.8-mile out-and-back

Elevation Range: 130' at the start to sea level

Facilities: Water, restrooms, and commercial facilities in the village of La Jolla

Highlights: One of California's most famous and dramatic meldings of land and sea

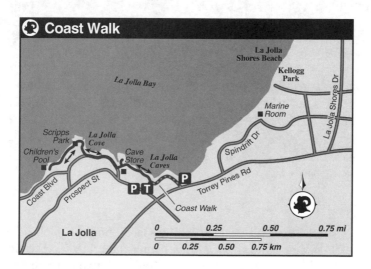

DESCRIPTION

You get a stunning perspective of La Jolla Bay and the sparkling La Jolla Shores coastline on this short walk along the clifftops. You'll be walking directly above the La Jolla Caves, on or near the very brink of a 100-foot drop to the bay's calm surface. This fact should alert you to be watchful of small children, if you have any along.

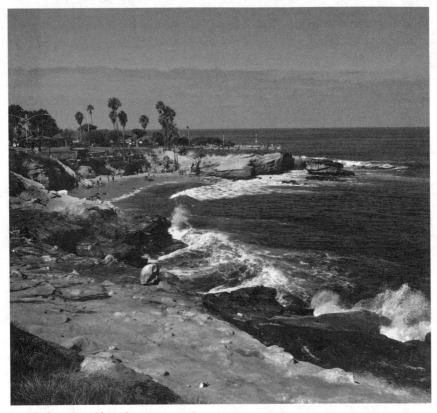

La Jolla Cove viewed from the east

THE ROUTE

From the Prospect Street cul-de-sac parking spaces, find the public access stairs and path leading toward a trail paralleling the brink. To the right, the trail leads a short distance over a wood bridge to two obscure public parking spaces at the west end of a paved street signed as Coast Walk (an alternative place to park your car). We turn left and pass below the back-yards of several palatial houses, all the while enjoying a spacious panorama of the blue ocean.

After only 0.2 mile, you arrive at a grove of graceful, planted Torrey pine trees. A fenced viewpoint lies below on the right, and The Cave Store, a designated City of San Diego Historic Landmark, lies immediately to the left. The whitewashed bluffs reflect large colonies of cormorants (Brandt's and double-crested) and brown pelicans that roost here. Adding to the quintessential SoCal atmosphere along this section, California sea lions bark and bellow from exposed rocks and ledges just beyond, while gulls wheel and call overhead. The Cave Store, which has gone by different names in the past and dates from 1902, features a 145-step staircase down a hand-carved tunnel leading to the westernmost of the series of La Jolla Caves— Sunny Jim Cave. There is a small fee per person to enter through the gift shop for a short descent to Sunny Jim Cave and its surf-kissed cavern.

Press on, continuing downhill on a sidewalk now, to the pocket beach of La Jolla Cove and the adjoining grassy space known as Scripps Park. Along the way, you can watch swimmers, snorkelers, and divers below as they float or glide through the often-glassy water. Once in Scripps Park, simply follow the curving sidewalk that stays close to the pounding surf, just below. After 5 or 10 minutes on the sidewalk, you'll arrive at the ever-popular Children's Pool breakwater and pocket beach, which has gained much attention over the years on account of its wholesale colonization by harbor seals.

After gawking at the seals, which are separated from the tourist crowds by a rope barrier, you can either head back the way you came, or try a different tack: head uphill, two blocks inland, to Prospect Street. Prospect Street is La Jolla's most elegant shopping-boutique thoroughfare, and it can take you straight back to your starting point.

TO THE TRAILHEAD
GPS Coordinates: N32° 50.877'   W117° 16.083'

From northbound I-5 (Exit 26A) or westbound CA 52 (Exit 1A), take La Jolla Parkway west toward La Jolla. La Jolla Parkway merges into Torrey Pines Road after 1.2 miles. Continue west on Torrey Pines Road another 1 mile to Prospect Street. Turn right, and within a short block, find the short cul-de-sac on the right with free public parking spaces. If this area is full, you may be able to find free parking on surface streets in this neighborhood or, occasionally, a bit farther west and down to the right along Coast Boulevard near The Cave Store.

23 Soledad Mountain

Trailhead Location: La Jolla

Trail Use: Hiking, dog walking, running, bicycling

Distance & Configuration: 5-mile out-and-back

Elevation Range: 100' at the start to 811' at the top of Soledad Park

Facilities: No restrooms along the route; portable restroom and drinking water in Soledad Park

Highlights: World-class coast-to-mountain vistas and residential mansions to admire

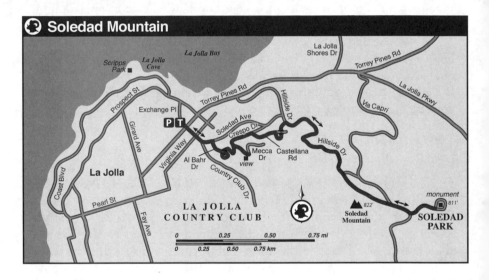

DESCRIPTION

Follow this eclectic route for a unique look at La Jolla, from the edge of the village's commercial center to 811 feet of elevation atop Soledad Mountain. Cyclists using road or mountain bikes can follow this same route, but beware: there are some tough uphill stretches here, suitable only for bikes with very low gears or a willingness to walk the bike in some spots. The Soledad Park vehicle gate is open daily, 7 a.m.–10 p.m.

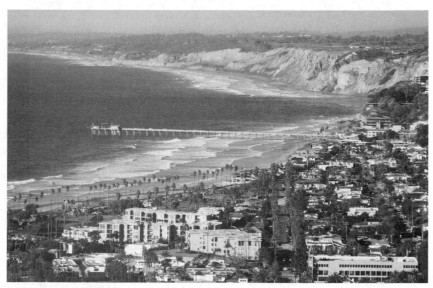

View of La Jolla Shores

THE ROUTE

Set off by going south (uphill) on Exchange Place. Busy Torrey Pines Road lies right ahead, and you may need to use the traffic light at Prospect, one block away, to cross safely on foot. Continue up Exchange Place and into one of La Jolla's serene older neighborhoods.

Within three short blocks, Exchange Place splits into Country Club Drive on the right and Soledad Avenue on the left. Take the left fork. After one block on Soledad Avenue, go right on Al Bahr Drive. On Al Bahr, follow a curious curlicue under and then over a gracefully arched bridge. At the top of the curlicue, turn right on Crespo Drive.

After completing a hairpin turn on Crespo, look for the intersection of Mecca Drive on the right. An optional but worthwhile side trip (that adds only 0.3 mile round-trip) to this 5-mile walk takes you higher up this dead-end narrow lane to a startling drop-off that offers airy and unobstructed views of La Jolla Bay and the North County coastline. Here, you can enjoy the same stupendous views afforded from some of La Jolla's finest homes.

Back down (or ahead, if you did not venture up Mecca Drive) on Crespo Drive, look for the inconspicuous intersection of Castellana Road, where you veer right. Just ahead, you can visit a hidden overlook at the point where Puente Drive, a stubby cul-de-sac, passes over Castellana Road on an arched bridge similar to the one seen earlier. From there, tall trees frame a view of tile rooftops and La Jolla Bay.

Next, back up a little and follow Castellana as it goes under the bridge and descends to meet Hillside Drive. Turn right on Hillside and follow its steep and winding course upward along the north slope of Soledad Mountain. Make no turns; just stay on the main winding drive, which is flanked by cliff-hanging mansions, some of them perched on postage stamp–size, outrageously expensive-view lots. In between these choice properties are jaw-dropping vistas of the coastline curving to the north.

On ahead you'll come to a sturdy, unlocked pipe gate. Go through it, maintaining your course upward on the old (now closed to traffic) roadbed of Hillside Drive. After some huffing and puffing and ever-widening views of the inland landscape, you reach Via Capri. From there you have only another 5 minutes or so of not-so-pleasant road-shoulder walking to reach Soledad Park.

A tall Easter cross still stands at the high point of Soledad Park, despite decades of controversy centered on the legality of its continued existence. A veteran's memorial installation now surrounds the cross to serve as a memorial to fallen soldiers and sailors.

The view from the base of the Easter cross is panoramic, except to the west where a slightly higher ridge—the true summit of Soledad Mountain—rises. In every other direction, you can check out the seemingly infinite spread of urbia/suburbia spreading east toward the distant mountain crest and the arterial pattern of wide freeways and major streets curving this way and that. In the south, skyscrapers in downtown San Diego loom, Mission Bay sparkles in the sunshine, and Point Loma juts like a southward pointing finger into the blue Pacific.

After enjoying the summit view, head back downhill, returning the same way you came.

TO THE TRAILHEAD
GPS Coordinates: N32° 50.770'   W117° 16.201'

From northbound I-5 (Exit 26A) or westbound CA 52 (Exit 1A), take La Jolla Parkway west toward La Jolla. La Jolla Parkway merges into Torrey Pines Road after 1.2 miles. Continue west on Torrey Pines Road another 1 mile to Prospect Street and turn right. Within a short block, turn left on Park Row. Park at or near the intersection of Park Row and Exchange Place, just ahead.

24 Marian Bear Memorial Park

Trailhead Location: Inland from La Jolla

Trail Use: Hiking, dog walking, running, mountain biking

Distance & Configuration: Up to 6.8 miles (double out-and-backs)

Elevation Range: 100'–240'

Facilities: Water, restrooms, and picnic tables at the start; restrooms and picnic tables near Regents Road parking

Highlights: Canopies of live oak and sycamore trees, plus a trickling stream; interpretive kiosks

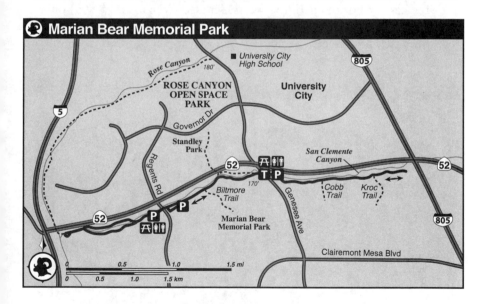

DESCRIPTION

Eastbound in the right lane of CA 52, the San Clemente Canyon Freeway, you can look down on a long, slender, almost unbroken swath of natural vegetation: massive sycamores, stately live oaks, climbing vines, and tangled shrubs. This is one of San Diego County's best examples of riparian (stream-loving) vegetation, and it's very rare in Southern California. Only 0.1% of San Diego County's land area consists of riparian vegetation.

Much of San Clemente Canyon and several of its steep finger (small tributary) canyons are included within the boundaries of Marian Bear Memorial Park, an area set aside by the city of San Diego as natural open space. Facilities include parking areas, picnic tables, and restrooms off Regents Road and Genesee Avenue and resting benches elsewhere. You won't get completely away from freeway traffic noise while hiking here, but you can minimize the disturbance by arriving early on Saturdays, Sundays, and holidays.

An old roadbed—today a trail of variable width—follows along the canyon's seasonal stream beneath the canopy of trees. The path stretches about 3 miles, is almost flat, and crosses the streambed four times. In summer these crossings simply mean a hop and a skip across cobblestones, but in winter some shallow-water wading may be necessary, typically at the first crossing east of Genesee and at the far west end.

The east end of the park (between Genesee Avenue and I-805) offers the prettiest vegetation, the densest shade, and a proliferation of poison oak vines that are adjacent to but not encroaching on the trail. Beginning

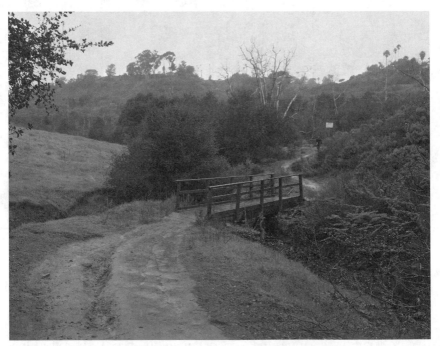

Bridge on Biltmore Trail on a rainy day

about October, the leaves of the poison oak turn bright red in pleasing complement to the evergreen live oaks and the yellows and oranges of the sycamores and willows. At other times of year these vines are leafless while the branches retain toxins to which many people have skin reactions. It is best to remain on the trails at all times to avoid contact and to help reduce impacts to vegetation.

THE ROUTE

Starting from the Genesee Avenue trailhead, you can travel as far as about 1 mile east toward I-805 or about 2 miles west toward I-5, all the while staying parallel to the freeway. That makes a round-trip of 6.8 miles if you go both directions.

In addition, a number of small side trails dart upward to hook up with neighborhoods to the north and south. Three south-trending side paths shown on the map are Kroc Trail, Cobb Trail, and Biltmore Trail (listed east to west). Each is worthy of exploration. Biltmore Trail features dense shade provided by coast live oaks and a small seasonal creek within narrow canyon walls. Taken together, these three provide 1 mile of bonus hiking.

Another side trail between the Genessee and Regents trailheads passes beneath CA 52 and ascends to Standley Park 0.5 mile to the north. At the west end of Marian Bear Memorial Park, a trail connects San Clemente Canyon to the next major open-space canyon area to the north, Rose Canyon Open Space Park.

TO THE TRAILHEAD

GPS Coordinates: N32° 50.749'   W117° 12.046'

Exit CA 52 at Genesee Avenue (Exit 2), which is 2 miles east of I-5 and 1 mile west of I-805. Go south on Genesee. The principal trailhead for Marian Bear Memorial Park is on the east side of Genesee, just south of the freeway. A U-turn on Genessee at the eastbound CA 52 on-ramp is necessary to access the entry gate. Gates are open daily, 5:30 a.m.–sunset.

25 Circling Sail Bay

Trailhead Location: Mission Beach

Trail Use: Hiking, running, dog walking, bicycling, in-line skating

Distance & Configuration: 5-mile loop

Elevation Range: Sea level up to 50' on major bridges

Facilities: A major commercial street, Mission Boulevard, lies one block west in the early part of the hike, so water and restrooms are handy at frequent intervals in the first half of the walk.

Highlights: A circumnavigation of picture-perfect, sail-flecked Sail Bay, the most scenic arm of Mission Bay

DESCRIPTION

More than a decade's worth of public improvements have literally paved the way for pedestrians, cyclists, Segway riders, and skaters traveling along the curving shoreline of west Mission Bay and its upper extremity, Sail Bay. Concrete paths, smooth enough for roller-skating but barely high enough to avoid being swamped at the highest tides, go right along the bay shoreline. To complete a loop around Sail Bay, you pass over open water three times via low-profile bridges on sidewalks that accompany busy roads. However, those sidewalks are generously wide and offer some fine views of the blue waters of Mission Bay and the colorful neighborhoods that surround it.

THE ROUTE

From your starting point at Dana Landing, follow the sidewalk going west toward West Mission Bay Drive. Some wooden stairs take you directly to the sidewalk that accompanies the roadway. Head west across the bridge over Mission Bay's main channel, and after another 0.5 mile veer right on Bayside Walk, a concrete pathway striking north along the shore of Mission Bay.

Bayside Walk differs enormously from the paralleling Ocean Front Walk, which borders the sand at Mission Beach only three blocks west. The popular Ocean Front Walk is often filled with cyclists, skaters, and pedestrians dodging each other, showing off, and gawking. If that's what you'd like to experience, then head over that way. Otherwise stay on the much more sedate Bayside Walk, which squeezes between wall-to-wall beach cottages on the left and the sandy shore of the bay on the right. You pass Santa Clara Point on the right, a popular launching spot for small sailing craft.

After more than a mile on Bayside Walk, you start curving east on newer and smoother slabs of concrete set low in the sand. Right after the Catamaran Resort, you gently climb and descend nearly 100 yards over the Briarfield Cove Bridge, spanning a tiny tidal slough at Sail Bay's north end.

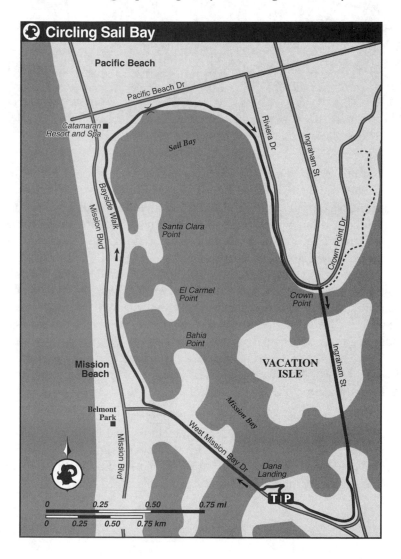

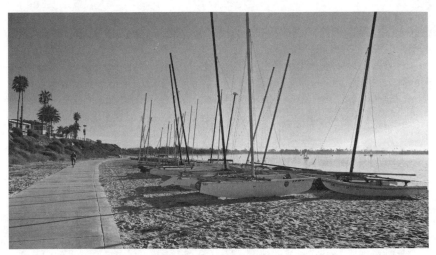
Catamarans on the beach

Continue curving past a grassy mini-park on the left and farther into Riviera Shores, which features multistory condominium buildings over-looking the water. When you reach the Ingraham Street Bridge, don't go straight under it but rather climb the stairway to the left, up to Riviera Drive at street level. Swing right on Ingraham Street and head south on Ingraham's sidewalk.

In the next mile, you pass over two long, separate bridges spanning Mission Bay, staying on the sidewalk all the while. These high points of the circuit provide your best opportunities to visually take in the total expanse of Sail Bay. On the far side of the second bridge, veer right toward Dana Landing Marina, and return to your parked car.

TO THE TRAILHEAD
GPS Coordinates: N32° 46.024'   W117° 14.346'

Exit I-8 at West Mission Bay Drive (Exit 1). Head north on a bridge over the San Diego River. As you approach the landscaped interchange ahead, go around the cloverleaf ramp to the right, following signs for the continuation of West Mission Bay Drive. Turn right at the first traffic light and park your car in any lot at or near the Dana Landing Marina.

26 Tecolote Canyon

Trailhead Location: East of Mission Bay

Trail Use: Hiking, dog walking, running, mountain biking

Distance & Configuration: Up to 6.5 miles out-and-back

Elevation Range: 50' at the start to 225'

Facilities: Water and restrooms at the start

Highlights: Pleasant springtime wildflowers and greenery

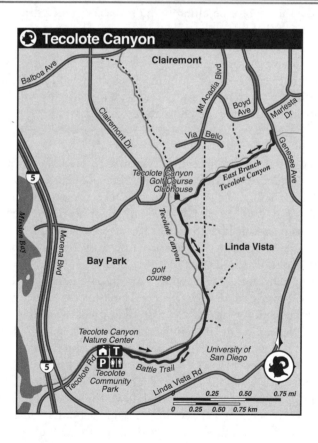

DESCRIPTION

The 900-acre Tecolote Canyon Natural Park knifes into two of San Diego's older and denser suburban neighborhoods, namely Clairemont and Linda Vista. World War II brought an initial building frenzy here, and intensive development continued into the 1970s. Like so many other places around San Diego, the canyon floor and its hillsides appeared to be slated for a major roadway and still more houses, but local advocates turned the tide and saved the canyon. Today, Tecolote Canyon is regarded as a valued habitat for native plants and animals and also welcomes anyone curious enough to visit.

On the natural park's patchwork of old roads and trails, it's possible to poke into just about every nook and cranny. By day you're sure to spot a hawk soaring on the thermals or perching high on the crown of a dead oak tree. By night you might hear the yapping of a coyote or the plaintive hoot of an owl, the creature for which this canyon was named.

For all but the most cursory exploration of this canyon, you should wear hiking boots or at least a pair of running shoes designed for off-road traction. Parts of the trail system are rough, but even small kids will like it—though perhaps not if they are forced to go too far.

THE ROUTE

Only the lower two-thirds of Tecolote's trail system is covered on our map. In addition to the primary trailhead next to the Tecolote Canyon Nature Center, the park has eight other neighborhood trail access points, and some of those are north of Balboa Avenue. The small, inviting nature center makes a great first stop for this hike. Maps, static displays, and announcements for upcoming special events are available here, as well as friendly park staff to answer your questions.

Here, we concentrate on the main, wide, smooth path going up Tecolote Canyon's broad lower end. The first mile is fine for casual walking, jogging, and mountain biking, at least at first. You can look at the sage scrub and chaparral vegetation in late winter and spring, when such plants are green and flowery. Down along the canyon's small stream channel, live oaks, willows, and sycamores thrive.

After about a mile, as you approach the perimeter of the Tecolote Canyon Golf Course, you'll start struggling up and down some steep hillsides. A narrow path on the left contours above the golf course, not far above the perimeter fence. It bends east on the slope overlooking the golf clubhouse and descends to an east branch of the canyon. The hike up along this fine,

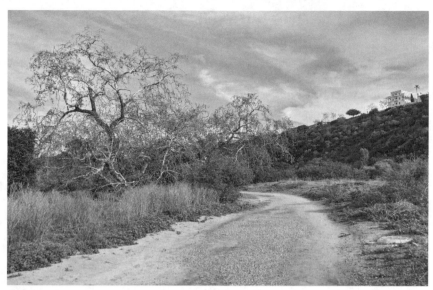

Trail in lower Tecolote Canyon

oak- and sycamore-dotted finger canyon to as far as Genesee Avenue is well worth it. If you reverse your steps upon reaching Genesee and return to the starting point, your round-trip hike measures about 6.5 miles. The upper section beyond the driving range along a tributary of Tecolote Creek may involve getting a bit wet as you navigate seven creek crossings along a twisting singletrack that at times dead-ends on spurs, especially in the upper 0.25 mile below Genesee Avenue. Watch out for abundant poison oak thriving here under the oak canopy—leaves of three, let them be.

Back in the lower canyon, consider exploring the Battle Trail on your left, a nice option for the return hike. It is tucked up against the south rim shortly after you pass a dirt access road leading up to the University of San Diego campus. Two signed junctions provide access to this shady, single-track bypass of the main trail—at 0.65 mile and 0.1 mile from the trailhead.

TO THE TRAILHEAD

GPS Coordinates: N32º 46.540'   W117º 11.842'

Exit I-5 at SeaWorld Drive/Tecolote Road (Exit 21). Drive 0.6 mile east on Tecolote Road to reach Tecolote Community Park and the nature center for Tecolote Canyon Natural Park immediately beyond.

27 San Diego River Channel— Ocean Beach

Trailhead Location: Ocean Beach/Dog Beach parking lot

Trail Use: Hiking, running, dog walking, biking, skating

Distance & Configuration: 4-mile out-and-back (up to 4.5 miles with side trips)

Elevation Range: Slightly above sea level throughout

Facilities: City beach amenities, Robb Field Recreation Center, and sports fields

Highlights: Postcard sunsets, wildlife preserve, starting point for San Diego River Trail

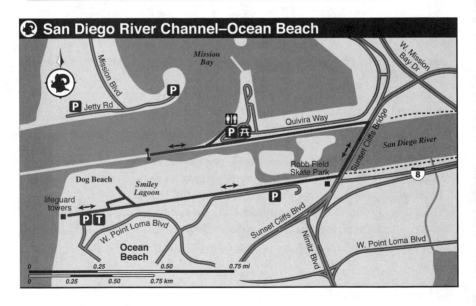

DESCRIPTION

Welcome to lands' end, a scenic delight at the westernmost point of the San Diego River Trail. Follow a nearly level bike path along two berms connected by Sunset Cliffs Boulevard Bridge over the San Diego River Channel, constructed decades ago to control rare, seasonal flooding of

San Diego's namesake river. Known worldwide as a birding hot spot, this saltwater/freshwater transition zone, known as the Southern Preserve, borders the southern portion of Mission Bay. This brackish estuarine habitat is refreshed twice daily by tides, providing food and shelter for countless resident and visiting waterfowl, shorebirds, and waders, many passing through on flights north or south along the Pacific Flyway. An osprey family has nested here for many years. The parents can often be seen diving and catching silvery mullet or other unsuspecting finny morsels to deliver to their ever-hungry—and begging—youngsters, with up to three chicks squeezed into their gigantic stick nest. The elusive light-footed Ridgway's rail might also be sighted but is more likely heard, and the endangered least tern may be spotted nesting here in nondescript scrapes in the sand. Come back regularly and you will likely see a host of new arrivals since your previous visit. Nearby Dog Beach is one of our region's most popular off-leash areas, and it is easy to see why—sand, surf, and acres of freedom. Stay for sunset and you might even catch the elusive green flash at the very instant the sun dips below the horizon.

Dogs are required to be on leash in all areas except on Dog Beach. Dogs are not allowed on the north trail November–March, 9 a.m.–4 p.m., and April–October, 9 a.m.–6 p.m.

THE ROUTE

Our start is from the City of San Diego parking area adjacent to Dog Beach. During the peak of summer, try to arrive early morning or late afternoon to guarantee finding a spot. Head north up a short ramping sidewalk to reach the trailhead and the stylistic Dog Beach surfboard marking the start. Turning left (west) takes you to the end of the path at Lifeguard Tower 5 that juts a short distance into the surf on both sides. Dogs and their owners frolic in spray to the right while surfers catch rides just off the south jetty that separates Mission Bay's entrance from the river channel. The shoreline to the south is for people only and provides one of San Diego's less crowded beach opportunities most of the year.

Turning back to the east, follow the multiuse path for just under 1 mile to Sunset Cliffs Bridge. It is possible to continue under the bridge following the San Diego River Trail as far as Mission Valley and beyond. This next section is a bit noisy with freeway traffic but does provide great birding and longer exercise options. Instead, we go up a short ramp and cross the bridge on the west sidewalk. You may see an osprey perched on a light pole while it surveys the water below for that next catch. On the far side of the bridge, turn left (west) and descend to another multiuse path and head as far west as you can go, typically the gated closure across from Dog Beach. A tidally driven "river" flows in and out close to the south-facing base of this jetty. On the north side, recreational vessels navigate an all-saltwater channel leading to Mission Bay. It is popular with fishermen too. At times of high surf and high tides, the outer reaches of this jetty can be awash, hence the gate. Though literally a stone's throw from Dog Beach, you have walked 2 miles to this point.

Return by the same route and appreciate a surprisingly different perspective, now looking inland toward Mission Valley and the mountains of the Peninsular Range, where the river begins. After crossing the bridge and passing the Robb Field complex, consider a short excursion on one of several sandy paths leading to low dunes inland from Dog Beach. Small interpretive signs identify resident species of plants and animals. If you were able to begin your hike in the afternoon, try adjusting your pace to arrive back at Life Guard Tower 5 a few minutes before sunset.

TO THE TRAILHEAD
GPS Coordinates: N32° 45.247'   W117° 15.095'

Take I-8 westbound until it terminates at Sunset Cliffs Boulevard and Nimitz Boulevard. Turn left (southwest) at this intersection and keep to the right lane on Sunset Cliffs for 0.5 mile. Turn right (west) at West Point Loma Boulevard and continue 0.5 mile toward the beach. Turn right (west) on Voltaire Street, and enter the large lot adjacent to Dog Beach; find a parking space wherever you can.

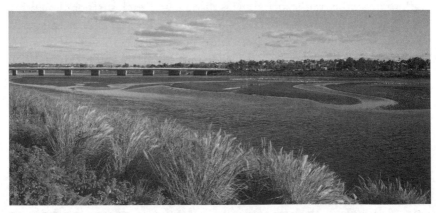

Sunset Cliffs Boulevard bridge

28 La Playa & Point Loma

Trailhead Location: Point Loma

Trail Use: Hiking, running, limited dog walking

Distance & Configuration: 2.5-mile loop

Elevation Range: Sea level to 170'

Facilities: The Point Loma business district is nearby.

Highlights: Fine homes and San Diego Bay and marina views

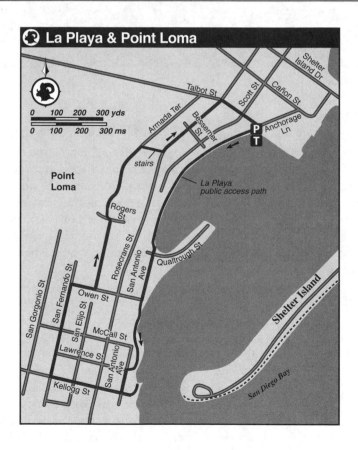

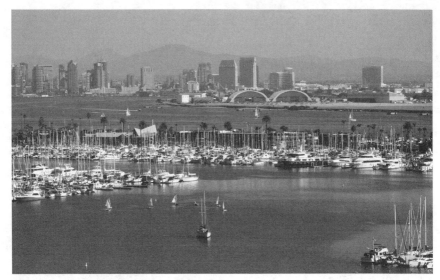

San Diego skyline from Armada Terrace

DESCRIPTION

This circular route follows a publicly accessible bayside pathway and rambles along narrow residential lanes in a San Diego Bay–facing neighborhood of Point Loma. Along the way, you'll pass two of the city's most celebrated marinas, the San Diego and Southwestern Yacht Clubs. Near the end, at an obscure opening between two hillside houses, you enjoy a view with a sense of déjà vu: the secret spot where local postcard photographers produce some of their most famous images. You can enjoy the bay-shore part of this ramble with your leashed dog too—but not 9 a.m.–5 p.m., when the path is closed to pets.

THE ROUTE

From Anchorage Lane, head down the sandy, bayside path. Shelter Island, to the left, fringed with yachts, extends nearly parallel with your path. The island is a peninsula, really—an artificial barrier island made of sand and mud dredged from the bottom of the bay. Some of San Diego's finest homes lie to your right, in the pocket neighborhood known as La Playa.

After about 0.5 mile, the bayside pathway joins San Antonio Avenue. Follow this residential street about three blocks, and when the pavement runs out, return to the shore, a sandy intertidal beach flecked with shells. Continue on to the end of that sandy stretch, where you approach the boundary fence of the Naval Base Point Loma, which occupies a big chunk of the Point Loma peninsula ahead. Simply turn right at that fence, and follow Kellogg Street west. Due to erosion, this one last short stretch of beach may be closed, in which case turn right at Lawrence Street and proceed south on San Antonio. A left turn at Kellogg leads to a small public beach at the harbor outlet, with the tip of Shelter Island just across the way. You may be tempted to dip your toes in the clear, calm waters here. Return to Kellogg Street heading away from the bay, cross Rosecrans Street, and continue uphill into one of Point Loma's most attractive and quiet residential areas.

Two blocks past Rosecrans, turn right on San Fernando Street. Pepper trees lining both sides of the street help conceal several opulent residences. Tall pines and eucalyptus trees reach into the sky, often snagging the cottony morning fog creeping over Point Loma's ridgeline. Check out the novel objets d'art placed in front of several of these homes, guaranteed to tease a smile.

A right turn on Owen Street followed by a left turn on San Elijo Street takes you to a T intersection at Rogers Street. Turn left (west) and walk about 30 feet to find a narrow, dirt pathway threading north between two homes. After a short passage, you'll reach the dead end of Armada Terrace. Follow Armada north toward Talbot Street, catching glimpses of the city, the bay, and the yacht basin. Many classic, long-lens photographs of San Diego's downtown skyline have been captured hereabouts, especially between two residential properties that happen to have a public stairway descending between them. From the top of that stairway, the panoramic view includes hundreds of boats at anchor, directly in front of a wide patch of San Diego Bay, plus the toothy downtown San Diego skyline.

Take that same public stairway down to Rosecrans, and turn left when you reach it. (If you overlook or pass the stairs, use the next street, Bessemer Street, to reach Rosecrans.) Head north to Talbot Street, turn right, and within two blocks you'll be back at your parked car.

TO THE TRAILHEAD
GPS Coordinates: N32° 43.146'   W117° 13.871'

From I-5 or I-8, at the interchange where the two freeways meet, take the Rosecrans Street exit (Exit 20). Proceed 3 miles southwest on Rosecrans to Cañon Street. Turn left, drive three blocks, and turn right on Anchorage Lane. Go one block and park on the street, where Anchorage Lane becomes Talbot Street. A commemorative plaque marks the start of a bayside pathway here.

29 Shelter Island

Trailhead Location: Point Loma

Trail Use: Walking, running, night hiking

Distance & Configuration: 2-mile out-and-back

Elevation Range: Sea level throughout

Facilities: Drinking water, public restrooms, hotels, and restaurants throughout

Highlights: Witness San Diego's best sunrises, sunsets, and moonrises from Shelter Island's shoreline pathway.

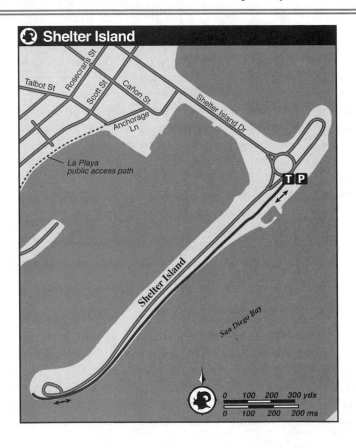

DESCRIPTION

If, as a San Diegan, Shelter Island seems overly familiar to you, then try visiting this artificial island (or shall we say peninsula, which is technically more correct) at either the opening or the closing of any clear day. That's when magic occurs with the sun, and sometimes the moon.

First, let's mention some of the island's history and its features. From its origins as a muddy shoal, the island was built up as dry land through dredging operations in San Diego Bay in the 1930s and '40s. By the 1950s, development was under way, and the island assumed its present persona as a shoreline resort destination, with hotels, restaurants, marinas, and a linear stretch of parkland about a mile long that features one of the finest walking paths in town. Over the years, several pieces of public art have been installed alongside that path. They include the *Tunaman's Memorial* (a bronze sculpture of tuna fishers in action), the *Yokohama Friendship Bell* (a gift from the city of Yokohama, Japan), and two monumental sculptures at opposite ends of the island—*Pacific Portal* and *Pearl of the Pacific*—by local artist James Hubbell.

Shelter Island's maritime eye candy includes hundreds of boats at anchor, most of which are associated with the Silver Gate, Southwestern, and San Diego Yacht Clubs. The shoreline is a favored spot for viewing Fourth of July fireworks over San Diego Bay and December's holiday lights boat parade.

From an astronomical standpoint, Shelter Island is visually sweet because it lies 3–4 miles due west of and straight across the bay from downtown San Diego's skyscrapers. Try taking a walk on the island path during either sunrise or sunset. In March and April, and also in September and October, the rising sun's rays thread through gaps between the distant buildings. The setting sun during those same months sends reflections off of any glass or metal surface in the downtown area, and the skyline burns with a fiery glow.

Every time there's a full moon, the moon's act of rising in the east is coincident (or nearly coincident) with the sun's setting. Again, for the months of March, April, September, and October, the rising full moon at sunset is closely aligned over the skyline. Barring low clouds or fog, the scene is a spectacle to behold.

THE ROUTE

From Shelter Island's traffic circle, on the side of the island facing downtown San Diego, pick up the shoreline sidewalk curving southeast past a public fishing pier. In the next 1 mile, enjoy the superlative views and walk along with all sorts of locals and tourists. Grassy spaces and picnic tables, all very popular for family get-togethers on fair-weather weekends, flank the sidewalk.

When you reach the far end of the island, turn around and return, enjoying the same great vistas from the reverse perspective.

TO THE TRAILHEAD

GPS Coordinates: N32º 43.008'   W117º 13.341'

From I-5 or I-8, at the interchange where the two freeways meet, take the Rosecrans Street exit (Exit 20). Proceed 3 miles southwest on Rosecrans to Shelter Island Drive. Turn left and drive 0.7 mile to the traffic circle on Shelter Island. Parking spaces are abundant either on the street or in the large public parking lots just past the traffic circle.

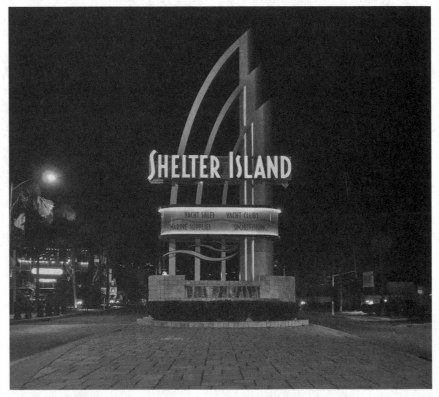

The sign at Shelter Island welcomes you.

30 Cabrillo National Monument

Trailhead Location: Tip of Point Loma

Trail Use: Hiking, running

Distance & Configuration: 2-mile out-and-back (Bayside Trail) and 1.5-mile out-and-back (Coastal Trail)

Elevation Range: 420' to sea level

Facilities: Water and restrooms at the adjacent Cabrillo National Monument Visitor Center

Highlights: The most comprehensive Pacific Ocean and San Diego Bay views you can get—short of flying—and a seaside walk on rugged cliffs above crashing Pacific waves

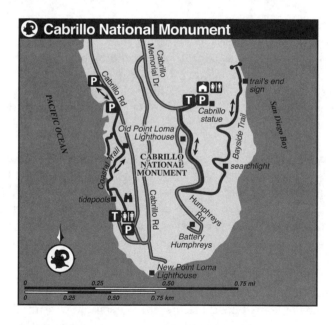

DESCRIPTION

The long, south-pointing peninsula of Point Loma and the spectacular curving shoreline of San Diego Bay are two of the principal elements responsible for San Diego's legendary beauty. Most of the south half of the

Point Loma peninsula is reserved for military uses. Perched on its end, centered on the highest promontory, is one of America's smallest (144 acres) national monuments, Cabrillo National Monument. Because of its location adjacent to the tourist-happy city of San Diego, Cabrillo is consistently ranked as one of the top 10 busiest national monuments in the country.

Hikers can enjoy the view-rich Bayside Trail that begins at the historic Old Point Loma Lighthouse atop Point Loma and offers an incomparable view of the city of San Diego and its watery environs. Amid the sweet-pungent sage scrub and chaparral vegetation, you get an eyeful of San Diego Bay, the Silver Strand, and the gleaming downtown skyline. You'll double your pleasure if you walk this trail on a crystal-clear day, fairly typical of the late-fall and winter seasons in San Diego. On the west side of the point, Cabrillo Coastal Trail provides dramatic contrast with colorful, eroded sandstone bluffs, booming surf, plus one of the best preserved tidepools in all of the San Diego region.

THE ROUTE

From the Cabrillo National Monument parking lot, first head south (uphill) to the lighthouse. Just east of the lighthouse, pick up the signed Bayside Trail, which begins with 0.3 mile of descending pavement. Make a hard left turn and travel the remaining 0.7 mile of gravel-surfaced trail. You descend east, losing most of the remaining elevation, and then turn north. Large metal interpretive plaques have been installed along this latter part of the trail, detailing the cultural and natural history of the area.

Point Loma's bay slope is honeycombed with the ruins of a World War II defense system of gun emplacements, observation and storage bunkers, generators, and searchlights. You will see some of these remains along the trail. At the point where the trail ends (or rather runs into off-limits U.S. Navy property), you'll still be about 90 feet in elevation above San Diego Bay's surface. This is a good place to observe the sailboats and ships maneuvering in and out of the bay's narrow entrance. There are also aerial acrobatics to watch, courtesy of gulls, terns, and pelicans—plus, possibly, aircraft taking off and landing at the North Island Naval Air Station across the bay.

Return to the lighthouse the same way you came, uphill all the way. Tempting as it may be, don't take shortcuts: the vegetation is easily trampled and the soil eroded by one footprint too many. Besides, off-trail exploration is strictly forbidden within the national monument.

Back at the Old Point Loma Lighthouse, consider taking a look inside, where you are allowed to climb partway up the spiral staircase. Not much

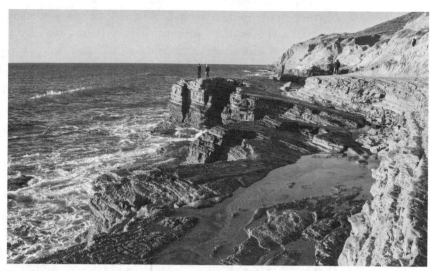

Pools below Cabrillo Coastal Trail

has changed appearance-wise from the structure's days as a working light-house, 1855–1891. Just south of the lighthouse, a whale-watching overlook offers a spectacular view west over what seems like the whole Pacific Ocean. December–February, migrating gray whales are commonly spotted swimming close to the shore. Binoculars help a lot in this endeavor.

If time permits, return to your car and drive down to the tidepool area on the west side of the monument. Starting just around the big bend and north of the "new" Point Loma Lighthouse (operating since 1891), the Coastal Trail zigs and zags for 0.75 mile along clifftops over and around deeply eroded sandstone ravines to the park's northern boundary. Unlike the Bayside Trail, here you can get down to the water and dip your toes in the Pacific at two places. During low tides you can also tour one of the richest tidepool communities San Diego has to offer.

If parking is available in the first lot, start from here. Otherwise try one of the other two lots, both on the left (west) side of Cabrillo Road. At the tidepool trailhead, volunteer interpreters staff an information table and can provide updates on tide times and share recent sightings. The tide-pools are reached following a short 0.15-mile walk—first north, then left down a few steps, then left again where a ledge-top path angles down to a cobble-covered cove. From late fall through early spring, extreme low tides occur here during daytime hours, exposing normally submerged rocks and ledges. Typical creatures you might see include skittering lined shore crabs and hermit crabs, Kellet's whelks, wavy turban snails, sea hares, brilliantly colored juvenile garibaldi (California's state fish) or Spanish shawl nudibranchs, and possibly an elusive octopus. Please don't pick up or disturb any of the tidepool critters or overturn rocks looking for them. Collecting of any kind is prohibited.

Doubling back to the main trail, continue north, following the winding trail to a series of close-to-the-edge vistas. A quarter mile ahead (0.4 mile from the start), a short, steep path descends wooden steps to another broad ledge less than 10 feet above the water where you are close to ever-pounding surf and spray. No extra charge for the saltwater showers! This area is popular with photographers, especially in the late afternoon when sun lights up these cliffs and backlights the spray. Watch your step here as extreme high tides can leave these ledges wet and slippery. Back up on top, the trail continues left (north) toward two other parking areas and higher vantage points for bird-watching or sighting spouts of migrating gray whales passing offshore to and from their winter breeding lagoons in Baja California. Return to your car via the same path.

Cabrillo National Monument closes at 5 p.m. year-round. Bayside Trail closes at 4 p.m., and the tidepool area and access road close at 4:30 p.m.

TO THE TRAILHEAD
GPS Coordinates:
Bayside Trail: N32º 40.438'   W117º 14.406'
Cabrillo Coastal Trail: N32º 40.094'   W117º 14.654'

From I-5 or I-8, at the interchange where the two freeways meet, take the Rosecrans Street exit (Exit 20). Proceed 3 miles southwest on Rosecrans to Cañon Street on the right. Drive uphill on Cañon Street, which merges with Catalina Boulevard after 1.2 miles. Keep going south on Catalina, past a military gate (open to the public from 9 a.m. to roughly sunset), and finally into Cabrillo National Monument at the road's end. Pay the fee at the entrance checkpoint, and head for the large parking lot beyond. To reach the tidepool area, turn right (west) just south of the entrance and go downhill on Cabrillo Road. There are three parking lots along the cliffs, with the first closest to the tidepools and trailhead. Due to safety concerns, pedestrian traffic on Cabrillo Road is discouraged.

31 Harbor Island

Trailhead Location: Next to San Diego International Airport

Trail Use: Hiking, running, dog walking, bicycling, night hiking

Distance & Configuration: 3.0-mile out-and-back (3.2 miles with loops at each end)

Elevation Range: Sea level throughout

Facilities: Drinking water, public restrooms, hotels, and restaurants throughout; self-pay rental bike stands

Highlights: Unbeatable bay and skyline views

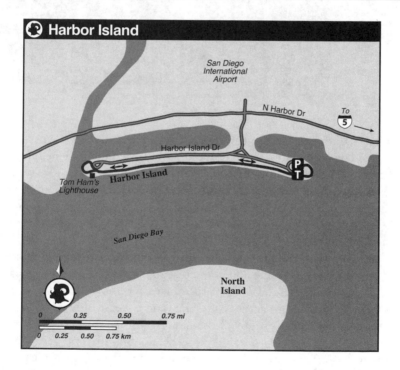

DESCRIPTION

Harbor Island, like Shelter Island (Hike 29, page 102), is an artificial, T-shaped peninsula lined with hotels, restaurants, small-boat marinas,

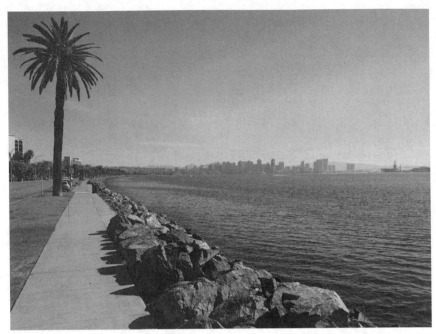

Morning skyline

and a grassy linear park fronting the waters of San Diego Bay. On the concrete sidewalk running the length of the linear park, you'll meet plenty of other people hanging out on benches, fishing from the sidewalk, watching for birds (which includes at least one resident great blue heron), and strolling or jogging along the path itself. Bikes and skates are not allowed on the path, though they are allowed to mix with the light car traffic on the adjacent roadway.

Almost any time of year and any time of day, the views from Harbor Island are at least handsome and at most stunning. Westbound, the panorama includes the Point Loma peninsula rising above the bay waters, aircraft carriers at anchor across the water, and a steady flow of large and small vessels cruising in or out of the bay. A whimsical mermaid sculpture graces the west end traffic circle. The eastbound vantage includes downtown San Diego's skyline, shadowy in the morning mist, gleaming in the golden light of afternoon, and often reflecting in the water. Behind the skyline, the higher mountaintops of San Diego County are visible on clear days. Off to the right, the San Diego-Coronado Bridge executes a low arc over the horizon.

THE ROUTE

Starting from Harbor Island's east end, follow the bayside sidewalk west. The gently curving sidewalk, flanked by benches and a grassy strip of variable widths, ends 1.5 miles later at Tom Ham's Lighthouse restaurant on the island's west end. To return, simply retrace your steps. With the right timing, you could face the setting sun on the outbound leg and the rising full moon on the return leg. As a variant to the main sidewalk, try out the short loop path encircling restaurants at the east end for gorgeous close-ups of the skyline. A similar loop around the parking lot at Tom Ham's takes you to the far west end of Harbor Island, with a view directly out to San Diego Harbor's entrance channel. Together these two loops add 0.2 mile to your route.

April–September, on nights when the moon is full, the rising moon appears right behind or nearly behind the skyline, particularly as seen from Tom Ham's. Savor the moment as the pumpkinlike moon silently launches itself right over the twilight-bathed city. (There is, however, one caveat about evenings on Harbor Island. Coastal San Diego commonly experiences May gray and June gloom. These seasonal low-overcast conditions spoil any view of the setting sun or rising moon.)

TO THE TRAILHEAD

GPS Coordinates: N32° 43.467'   W117° 11.373'

From I-5 just north of downtown San Diego, follow the signs for San Diego International Airport (Exit 18A, Sassafras Street/San Diego Airport). Signs will direct you onto westbound North Harbor Drive: 0.4 mile from the exit, merge into Kettner Boulevard for 0.8 mile, then turn right (west) on Laurel Street. In 0.3 mile, Laurel Street merges into North Harbor Drive. Stay in the leftmost lane (right lanes go into the airport) for 1.1 miles and turn left on Harbor Island Drive. Proceed 0.3 mile to where Harbor Island Drive splits east and west. Turn left (east) and drive to a spacious, free public parking lot at the end of the road, 0.5 mile ahead, or along one of the turnouts along Harbor Island Drive. The east parking lot is paid valet only after 4:30 p.m.

32 The Embarcadero

Trailhead Location: Downtown San Diego

Trail Use: Hiking, running, dog walking, bicycling

Distance & Configuration: 3-mile balloon

Elevation Range: Sea level throughout

Facilities: Everywhere along the route

Highlights: Bay and city vistas from San Diego's front porch

DESCRIPTION

San Diego's Embarcadero, the place of departure and arrival for vessels as small as fishing skiffs and as large as ocean liners, defines the city's connection to the watery worlds of San Diego Bay and the Pacific Ocean. The unquestionably spectacular views are somewhat marred by a preponderance of all-too-wide thoroughfares given over to car traffic, parking lots, and hulking military buildings.

All that is changing and will evolve over the next decades as several major redevelopment projects come online to spiff up the waterfront with wide walkways, grassy parks for picnics and entertainment events, more restaurants and retail outlets, and a remade skyline immediately inland. Therefore, our directions for travel along the Embarcadero will remain somewhat tentative for years to come.

THE ROUTE

A good starting place is the winding concrete sidewalk that follows the bay shoreline just north of the traffic lights at North Harbor Drive and Hawthorn and Grape Streets. To your right, modest sailing vessels of all stripes are moored. On a rotating basis, the Port of San Diego sponsors various artworks, such as *Bench Party*, wood and steel sculptures that allow visitors to enjoy the expansive views.

As you stroll south, the sidewalk widens, and you pass the collection of antique watercraft comprising the Maritime Museum of San Diego. The museum's signature attraction, the 1863 iron-hulled sailing vessel *Star of India*, currently qualifies as the world's oldest sailing ship still in regular use. Occasionally she can be seen tooling around San Diego Bay. Other vessels can be explored at their piers (with paid admission), and some can

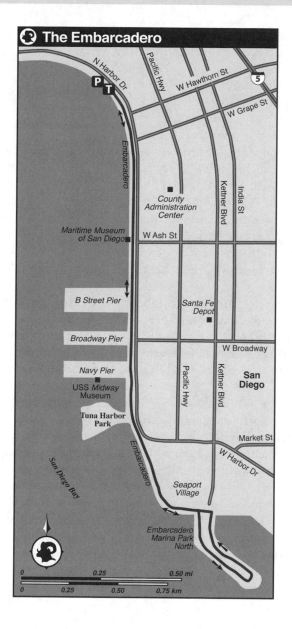

The Embarcadero

be boarded for sailing or powered cruises, such as the tall ship *Californian* (a replica of an 1847 revenue cutter) and a replica of Juan Rodriguez Cabrillo's *San Salvador*, the first European vessel to reach America's West Coast and the port of San Diego in 1542.

Next, on the bay side, are three major piers. The B Street Pier for cruise ships allows no pedestrian access. The Broadway Pier, an auxiliary terminal for cruise ships, allows pedestrians when ships aren't docked there. Small docks on either side of the Broadway Pier host vessels carrying tourists on bay excursions and whale-watching expeditions. Navy Pier, the southernmost of the three, serves as a parking lot for the USS *Midway* aircraft carrier (now a museum), which is permanently berthed there.

After Navy Pier, the sidewalk promenade widens to include Tuna Harbor Park. If you are inclined, take a short side trip over to see various public art exhibits with World War II themes. The park also has a viewpoint where you can look straight west toward the modern aircraft carriers at anchor alongside the Naval Air Station North Island. On the southwest side of Tuna Harbor Park lies a slightly gritty pier for commercial fishing boats. Walk out there to get a flavor for the San Diego working waterfront, complete with nets being repaired by commercial fishermen and lobster traps.

Resuming your travel south, you're quickly immersed in tourist heaven, with the shops and restaurants of Seaport Village on the left and a smooth whitewashed wall on the right, where you can sit and contemplate the whole of San Diego Bay's south arm, flecked with sailboats on windy days. The graceful arch of the San Diego–Coronado Bridge vaults over the scene.

Make a fitting end to your Embarcadero hike by following the looping sidewalk around the north section of Embarcadero Marina Park, just south of Seaport Village. The 360-degree vista from this grassy space encompasses the bay, a small-boat harbor jammed with pleasure craft, swanky hotels, and the nautically themed San Diego Convention Center. Embarcadero Marina Park hosts a variety of events throughout the year, including vintage car shows. Many families arrive early for traditional Fourth of July picnics and stay for evening fireworks synchronized to music that's broadcast over local radio. Whatever the day, you will likely find kindred souls enjoying some of the best harborside experiences that San Diego has to offer.

When you return to Seaport Village, simply retrace your earlier steps back to your starting point.

TO THE TRAILHEAD
GPS Coordinates: N32° 43.526'   W117° 10.440'

On North Harbor Drive, fronting San Diego Bay, and as close to West Hawthorn Street as possible, find any metered parking place or pay parking lot, or if you're lucky, one of a handful of free parking sites. This area is the recommended starting point because parking tends to be more available.

The closest freeway access is from I-5. If southbound, take the Sassafras Street/San Diego Airport exit (Exit 18A) and proceed 1.5 miles on Kettner Boulevard to Hawthorn, then head right (west) on Hawthorn 0.2 mile to Harbor Drive. If northbound, take the Hawthorn Street exit (also signed for San Diego Airport; Exit 17A) for 0.4 mile to merge into Hawthorn, passing beneath I-5, and go another 0.4 mile west to Harbor Drive.

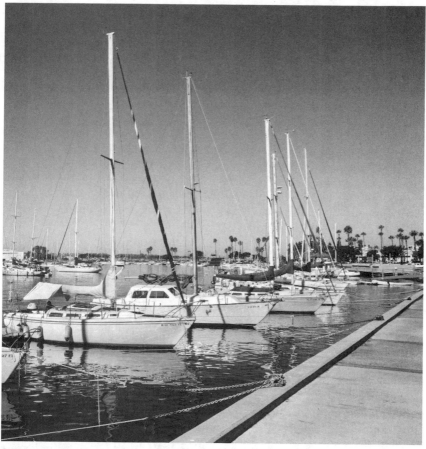

Sailboats along the Embarcadero

33 Bankers Hill

Trailhead Location: Just north of downtown San Diego

Trail Use: Hiking, dog walking, running

Distance & Configuration: 2.3-mile balloon

Elevation Range: 80' at the start to 290' in Bankers Hill

Facilities: One restaurant/store midway into the hike

Highlights: Historic houses and century-old footbridges

DESCRIPTION

With its quaint footbridges spanning two wooded ravines, scores of historic homes, plus a wealth of mature landscaping, Bankers Hill speaks to historical elegance and the preservation of nature. The following short ramble through canyon bottom and along quiet city streets takes you there—north and south, top and bottom.

THE ROUTE

From the end of Maple Street, make your way on foot up the wide, smooth path in the canyon bottom ahead, noting the mix of native sage scrub and chaparral vegetation and the nonnative eucalyptus trees and palm trees, the latter giving plenty of shade.

At about 100 yards into the canyon, notice the steep slope to the right. At the top, on the canyon rim, lies a historical marker commemorating the 1909 aviation feats of 15-year-old Waldo Waterman, who sailed off this perch on a homemade contraption and glided into the canyon bottom without breaking his neck. Waldo was still flying as a commercial pilot in 1959 when the dedication ceremony was held. The plaque, up at the corner of Albatross and Maple Streets, is better suited for a drive-by visit than a side trip climb on foot.

Farther up the canyon floor, you pass under the tall and graceful First Avenue Bridge, erected in 1931 and upgraded to modern engineering standards in 2009. After nearly 0.5 mile, you reach the wooden supporting beams of the equally historic Quince Street footbridge. A steep path through eucalyptus trees on the left connects to Third Avenue and houses above via log stairs. Trudge upward and make a right on Third Avenue.

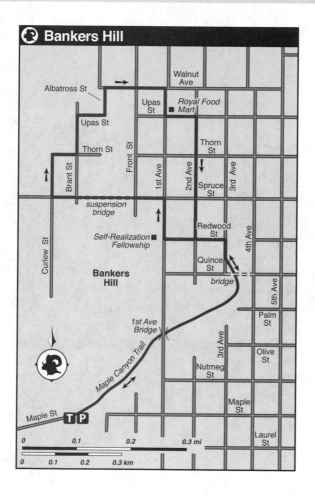

After only a half block, turn left on Redwood Street, and continue two blocks to First Avenue. You're now squarely in the historic Bankers Hill neighborhood, where many of the city's elite resided a century ago. Once you reach First, gaze across the street to spot the Self-Realization Fellowship, formerly Bishop's School (1909), partially designed by San Diego's renowned architect Irving Gill. The Gill-designed wing wraps around an older Tudor-style structure and epitomizes Gill's philosophy of simplicity and, as described by one of his critics, "monastic severity."

From Redwood and First, continue north on First Avenue to Spruce Street. (In case you hadn't noticed, east-west streets are ordered alphabetically from Ash and Beech in downtown San Diego to Redwood and

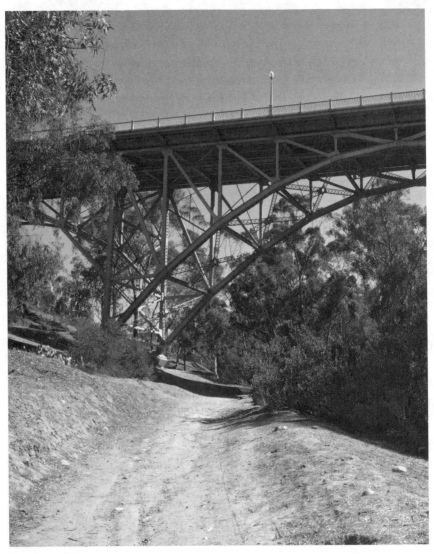

First Avenue Bridge

Spruce and beyond in Bankers Hill.) Make a left on Spruce Street and head west (downhill) to cross the 1912 Spruce Street suspension footbridge over a ravine commonly known as Arroyo Canyon. Pause in the middle of the swaying bridge, 70 feet above the canyon floor, and feel the breeze sweeping upcanyon from the bay.

On solid ground again at Brant Street, continue west another block to Curlew Street and turn right—all the while taking note of the varied architectural styles of the homes, most of which date back to the early 20th century. Many of the properties display historical plaques indicating the date of original construction.

Heading north on Curlew, you soon make a right on Thorn Street. Zigzag east on Thorn, north on Brant Street, east on Upas Street, and north on Albatross Street. On the east side of Albatross are some of Irving Gill's noted canyon houses, dating from 1912–13 and designed to blend harmoniously with the natural landscape of the ravine below. From Albatross, make a right on Walnut Avenue and proceed two blocks to First Avenue. Turn right and within a short block reach the Royal Food Mart, a restaurant housed in a circa 1930s structure whose exterior appearance and interior furnishings are suggestive of that time in history. Take a break for food or beverages here if you like. A reasonably priced deli with vintage furnishings, formerly a butcher shop serving this area for early 20th-century Bankers Hill residents, is accessed from the north door. The entrance to the adjacent sit-down café is closest to the street corner.

From the restaurant, go one block east on Upas Street to Second Avenue, and turn right. Enjoy the grand old homes in the next three blocks ahead. When you reach Redwood, go left for a block, turn right on Third Avenue, and finally make your descent into Maple Canyon, retracing your former route in the canyon bottom and back to your starting point.

TO THE TRAILHEAD
GPS Coordinates: N32° 43.940'   W117° 10.052'

Exit northbound I-5 at Hawthorn Street (Exit 17A) toward San Diego Airport. After merging into Hawthorn, turn right (north) immediately at State Street and follow it 0.4 mile, passing under I-5. Turn right (east) at West Maple Street. This segment of Maple Street ends two blocks east at a sign indicating Maple Street Open Space. Curbside parking is available on Maple or Dove Street.

34 Balboa Park's Central Mesa

Trailhead Location: Central Balboa Park

Trail Use: Hiking, running, dog walking

Distance & Configuration: 3-mile loop

Elevation Range: 220'–300'

Facilities: Water and public restrooms near the middle of the route

Highlights: Rose and succulent gardens, historic buildings and plazas, crossing the high Cabrillo Bridge

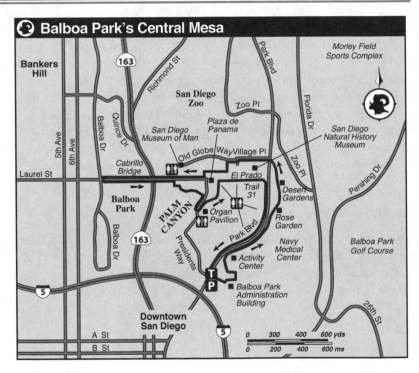

DESCRIPTION

Balboa Park's historic buildings, museums, gardens, and the world-famous San Diego Zoo have pretty much framed the site's reputation for decades. What many visitors and even locals don't know is that Balboa sprawls over a total of 1,200 acres, or nearly 2 square miles. That's a lot of space to explore for the self-propelled traveler.

Incremental improvements have taken place over the past several years throughout Balboa Park's hidden spaces. Canyon slopes formerly choked with weedy undergrowth and once used as drug dens have been cleared out and made user-friendly and safer for local residents and tourists. Forgotten pathways have been reconstructed, and new landscaping has been installed. As part of this process, the park has established five trail gateways (trailheads) and at latest count 19 marked trail routes that serve every corner of the park.

Balboa Park's Central Mesa incorporates two historical sectors: the 1915–16 Panama-California Exposition site on the north and the 1935–36 California Pacific International Exposition site on the south. Both expositions were fielded by the city of San Diego, then relatively small, for the purpose of gaining international attention. As in the case of nearly all world's fairs, the theme buildings hastily constructed for both expositions found later uses, such as housing museums and a variety of civic and cultural organizations.

The 1915–16 exposition site in particular is renowned among San Diegans for its incomparably beautiful Spanish-Moorish buildings, its gardens, and the graceful Cabrillo Bridge. That area is therefore the primary destination of this short hike. You'll be following signs for Trail 31 throughout.

THE ROUTE

From the Park Boulevard Gateway sign, first head east on the sidewalk leading directly toward the Balboa Park administration building. Climb the stairs, swing left around the headquarters building, and enjoy the pergola-bounded courtyard behind it. Comparatively few people visit this beautiful space.

From the courtyard, walk north and edge by the Balboa Park Activity Center (table tennis, badminton, volleyball, and the like are practiced inside). You emerge along the sidewalk following Park Boulevard. Continue north along the fenced perimeter of the Naval Medical Center San Diego. After a short distance you come upon the spacious Rose Garden and, just past that, the Desert Garden, a hillside covered with exotic succulent plants from around the world.

At the far north end of the Desert Garden, you arrive at the intersection of Park Boulevard and Village Place. Cross Park Boulevard at the traffic light there, and head west past the massive Moreton Bay fig tree that stands in front of the entrance to the San Diego Natural History Museum.

At the next street crossing, jog slightly left and pick up Old Globe Way on the far side. You skirt the south boundary fence of the San Diego Zoo for a short while, and then turn left, just short of the lath Botanical Building. Bear right alongside the front entrance to the Botanical Building, passing right over the majestically serene Lily Pond. Need we remind you to bring your camera?

Just ahead, you reach the park's central square, Plaza de Panama, bounded by two art museums on the north and various historical structures dating from the 1915–16 exposition on the south. The plaza was transformed into a popular pedestrian-only gathering space in time for the exposition's centennial in 2015. Featuring seating, shade umbrellas, and cultural delights around its perimeter, Plaza de Panama brings an old-world ambience to the heart of Balboa Park.

Following Trail 31 signs (which are plaques embedded in the sidewalk within the park's historical zones), continue west along El Prado, past the Museum of Man's lofty California Tower (tickets are available in the museum for a breathtaking tour to the viewing deck of the tower). Continue ahead all the way across the Cabrillo Bridge, using the northside sidewalk. The 450-foot-long, 120-foot-high bridge, begun in 1912, uses a multiple-arched cantilever structure, which was innovative at that time and timeless in its form.

At the far side of the bridge, cross over the El Prado roadway and pick up the southside sidewalk for the reverse direction (east). The historic Cabrillo Freeway (better known as the 163 freeway) curves below, leading toward the cluster of high-rises that defines San Diego's downtown skyline. Many a classic postcard photo was taken from this vantage.

Returning to the California Tower, veer right just ahead for a passage through peaceful Alcazar Garden and edge along the lushly landscaped upper rim of Palm Canyon. You then curve left toward the Organ Pavilion, which houses one of the world's largest pipe organs. Travel north from there past the Japanese Friendship Garden, and return to Plaza de Panama.

Make a right now, and go east on the traffic-free section of El Prado, passing museums on both sides. Continue all the way to the circular Bea Evenson Fountain. Finally, make your way down to the westside sidewalk on Park Boulevard, swing right, and follow that sidewalk back to the corner of Park Boulevard and Presidents Way, your starting point.

TO THE TRAILHEAD

GPS Coordinates: N32° 43.536'   W117° 9.015'

From downtown San Diego, follow Park Boulevard (12th Avenue) north. Right after passing over I-5, make a right at the first traffic light, Presidents Way.

From southbound CA 163, take the Park Boulevard exit (Exit 1B) shortly before CA 163 ends in downtown San Diego. Once on the transition ramp, follow the Park Boulevard signs while avoiding the far right lane (leading to I-5 North) and the far left lane (leading to I-5 South). At the Park Boulevard traffic light, turn left and continue to the next traffic light, Presidents Way. Park your car in one of the spacious lots near that intersection or along Park Boulevard itself. The Park Boulevard trail gateway sign is located at the northeast corner of Park Boulevard and Presidents Way.

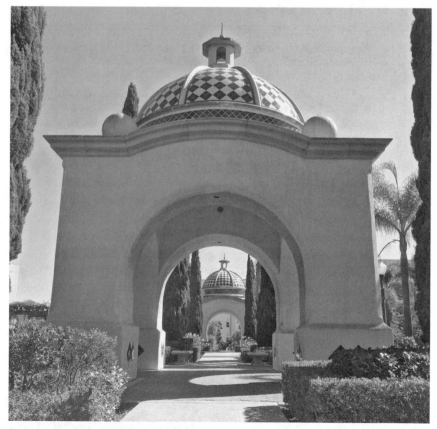

Arched domes in the courtyard

35 Balboa Park's East Side

Trailhead Location: Just east of downtown San Diego

Trail Use: Hiking, dog walking, running

Distance & Configuration: 4.4-mile loop

Elevation Range: The route goes up and down several times, staying between 100' and 340' of elevation.

Facilities: Water and restrooms at the start and at Morley Field Sports Complex, midway through the hike

Highlights: Explore Balboa Park's far-east quarter, beautifully landscaped in places and home to several unsung attractions.

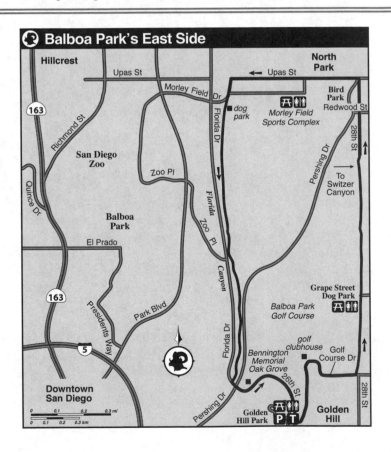

DESCRIPTION

Balboa Park's easternmost section isn't well known among most San Diegans, let alone tourists. Local residents, along with local golfers, do know of several out-of-the-way features here: Golden Hill Park, Balboa Park Golf Course, Grape Street Dog Park, Switzer Canyon, and Bird Park. Exploring this spacious area is the goal of this hike, which follows Trail 22 in the Balboa Park trails system. You'll be on a combination of unpaved trails (some briefly steep and rocky), sidewalks, and roadside shoulders.

THE ROUTE

Starting from the Golden Hill Park trail gateway sign, head east and slightly downhill from 25th Street to the four-way stop sign at 26th Street. Go straight across to Golf Course Drive, and stay on the left (west) wood-chip-surfaced shoulder of that two-lane road. Follow the road as it curves past the golf course clubhouse. Look behind to catch an unusual (if you haven't been in these parts before) vista of the downtown San Diego skyline.

Past a couple more curves, Golf Course Drive intersects with 28th Street. Very near that intersection, make a left on the signed trail heading due north. This sign is small and brown on a waist-high post, not one of the colorful Balboa Park trail signs. It faces south toward the street and is a few feet before a street signpost. Due north you go, paying no heed to the topography, down one steep hill and up another slope to flat land again. You go by the Grape Street picnic area and dog park on the left, only one of three areas within Balboa Park where unleashed dogs can roam.

Continue following the north-heading Trail 22, losing elevation again. You find yourself right alongside one of the golf course's fairways, fringed with a beautiful grove of planted native live oaks. Just ahead on the right you'll see an informational signboard for the Switzer Canyon Open Space, a small city-owned natural area occupying the canyon on the right side. Keep going straight, though, steeply uphill, and hook up with 28th Street on the rim of Switzer Canyon, staying to the right of the golf course.

Use the sidewalk of 28th Street to travel north for five blocks to Upas Street, passing numerous homes of historical importance. Notice the contractor's date stamps in the sidewalk concrete slabs. Bird Park, a mini-park within Balboa Park at 28th and Upas Streets, pays homage to San Diego's great variety of native birds.

Now head west on Upas Street for 0.5 mile, hang a left on Morley Field Drive, continue about 100 yards, and hang a left again at the entrance to a parking lot next to the Morley Field Dog Park. Travel south through the dog park and pick up the trail descending into Florida Canyon, Balboa

Park's primary area of native vegetation. At first glance the natural vegetation of Florida Canyon may appear scruffy and desiccated by comparison with the lushly (but artificially) landscaped acres of Balboa Park proper. The aesthetic differences between the two are minimized in late winter and early spring when new growth burgeons, sage and other aromatic plants emit sweet fragrances, and wildflowers carpet the ground.

Keep heading south, on the left (east) side of Florida Drive and more or less parallel to it, for just over 1 mile. You then reach the intersection of Pershing Drive, Florida Drive, and 26th Street on the far side. Use the pedestrian crosswalks and walk signals to get across to 26th Street, a curving road leading upward. Follow the right shoulder of the road, which doubles as the final leg of Trail 22. On the lower half of this climb, take note of the beautiful grove of live oaks arching over you, called the Bennington Memorial Oak Grove. Its trees were planted in memory of the more than 60 men killed in the boiler steam explosion that took place aboard the USS *Bennington* gunboat in San Diego harbor in 1905.

TO THE TRAILHEAD
GPS Coordinates: N32º 43.181'   W117º 8.415'

From Broadway or Market Street, the two main east-west streets in downtown San Diego, travel east to 25th Street (east of I-5), turn left, and go north to where 25th Street ends at Golden Hill Park (about 0.5 mile). Park for free in Golden Hill Park or on city streets. Look for the blue Balboa Park trail gateway signboard at the far north end of 25th Street. The closest freeway exit is CA 94 westbound to 25th Street (Exit 1B), then go right (north) on 25th for 0.4 mile to Golden Hill Park.

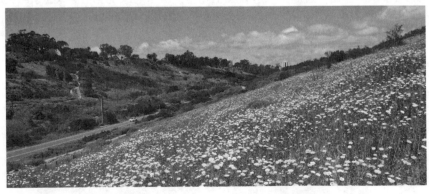

Chrysanthemums in Florida Canyon

36 Gaslamp Quarter

Trailhead Location: Downtown San Diego

Trail Use: Hiking

Distance & Configuration: 1-mile loop

Elevation Range: Near sea level throughout

Facilities: Water, restrooms, dining, and shopping plentiful along route

Highlights: San Diego's best historical scenery by day and the city's most vibrant nightlife

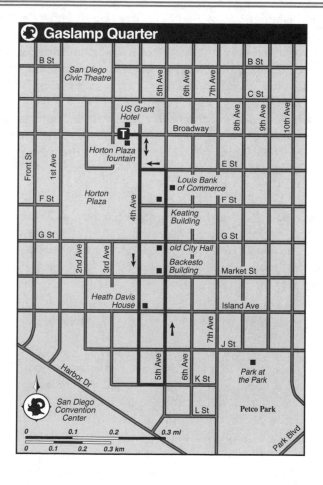

DESCRIPTION

Formerly San Diego's skid row, this core downtown historic area was reborn in the 1980s under a new name: the Gaslamp Quarter. Actually, gas lamps were never used for outdoor lighting in San Diego, though today you can find a few decorative ones. Rather, the district's distinctive gas lamp–style electric streetlights inform you whether you're in the Gaslamp Quarter or not. This is the place to go in the daytime for scoping out dozens of historic buildings dating from the late 1800s through the early 1900s and (by night especially) for feeling the pulse of thousands of visitors milling about, drinking at watering holes, and dining in fine restaurants.

Ignoring small exceptions, the Gaslamp Quarter stretches two blocks from west to east (Fourth and Sixth Avenues) and eight blocks from north to south (Broadway to Harbor Drive). The cheek by jowl pattern of buildings in the Gaslamp is unique among all San Diego neighborhoods. The frontages range from a narrow 25 feet to a broad 225 feet. The latter is the case for one historic site, the 1873 Backesto Building on Fifth Avenue at Market Street. You'll see modern (21st-century) architecture, but even that was designed to fit in harmoniously with the earlier structures. Added attractions at the margins of Gaslamp Quarter include Petco Park, two blocks to the east and home to the San Diego Padres Major League Baseball team, and the San Diego Convention Center, directly south across Harbor Drive where costumed intergalactic creatures and superheroes converge in July for the annual Comic-Con International event.

THE ROUTE

A definitive starting point for our Gaslamp Quarter tour is the historic Horton Plaza fountain at Fourth Avenue and Broadway. The century-old fountain was one of the first to combine colored lighting effects with flowing water. Across Broadway lies the elegant hotel The US Grant, dating from 1910. Immediately to the south, just outside the entrance to Horton Plaza shopping center, kids of all ages take their chances dashing through a 21st-century fountain featuring synchronized jets of water shooting up from the pavement.

Head south from either fountain on Fourth Avenue, staying on the left (east) side to remain close to a long row of historic buildings. More than 90 buildings throughout the Gaslamp are tagged with brass plaques, each including a short historical description. At the end of the fifth block (Fourth and Island Avenues), on the left, pay a visit to the William Heath Davis House (1850), the location of the Gaslamp Quarter Historical Foundation's visitor center. There you can pick up a guide map for the historic

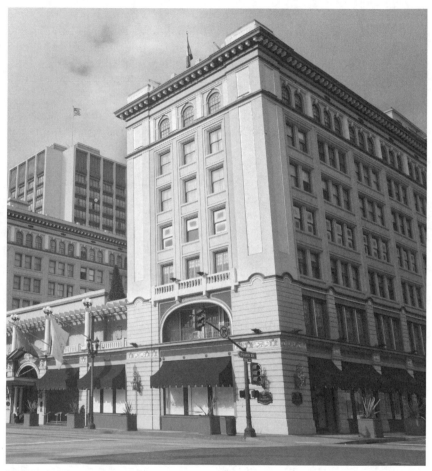

US Grant hotel

buildings in the Gaslamp district. Volunteer docents in period costumes lead tours of the two-story interior. You might even meet Alonzo Horton, father of San Diego, or Wyatt Earp, gambler, saloonkeeper, and business-man who resided during this period just across the street in the former Grand Horton Hotel (now the stylish Horton Grand Hotel).

After traveling two more blocks south (nearly as far as Harbor Drive and the convention center), swing left on K Street and left again on Fifth Avenue. The iconic Gaslamp Quarter sign arches enticingly over Fifth one block south at L Street. Now, as you head north on either side of Fifth, you're going to encounter the very best in historic architecture, or the wildest nightlife, assuming you're here during the late-night hours. Notable daytime sights include the old San Diego City Hall building (1874) at Fifth Avenue and G Street, the Backesto Building (the long, low one) at Fifth and Market Street, the 1890 Keating Building at Fifth and F Street, and the ornate 1888 Louis Bank of Commerce building on Fifth between E and F Streets. When you reach E Street, head back to Fourth to return to Horton Plaza.

Naturally, you'll be tempted to stray off of the route described above. You can head west to check out San Diego's tiny Asian district centered at Third and Island, head south to follow the arrow-straight path through the Martin Luther King Jr. linear park paralleling Harbor Drive, or skip a few blocks east and picnic at the grassy Park at the Park, which is adjacent to the Petco Park baseball stadium.

TO THE TRAILHEAD
GPS Coordinates: N32° 42.935'   W117° 9.692'

Drive to the Horton Plaza shopping center bounded by Broadway, Fourth Avenue, G Street, and First Avenue in downtown San Diego. For the closest freeway access from the merge of CA 163 southbound to I-5, take the Fourth Avenue exit (Exit 1B) and proceed south on Fourth to Horton Plaza (about 0.5 mile). Park in the parking garage of the shopping center (up to 3 hours validated free parking). Or try to find a parking space (free on Sundays) along any downtown street or in any pay parking lot near Horton Plaza. Start your walk at the historic Horton Plaza fountain on Broadway at Fourth Avenue or at any point along the route near where you parked.

37 Coronado Beach

Trailhead Location: Coronado

Trail Use: Hiking, running, dog walking, night hiking

Distance & Configuration: 3.8-mile out-and-back

Elevation Range: Sea level all the way

Facilities: Access to water and public restrooms near the middle of the beach; Coronado's commercial district lies a few blocks east.

Highlights: An extraordinarily wide beach packed with fine-grain sand, and with a glorious view of Point Loma and the ocean

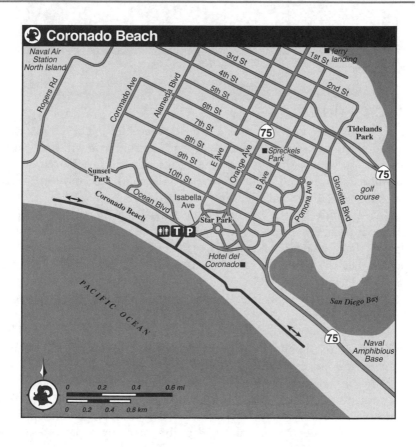

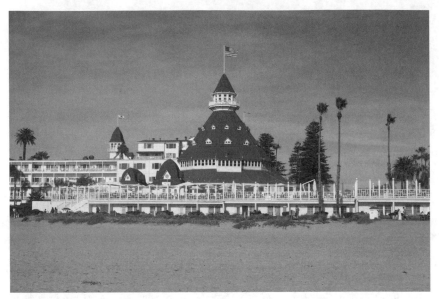

Hotel del Coronado

DESCRIPTION

Travel magazines routinely rank Coronado's oceanfront beach as one of the nation's most beautiful stretches of coastline, and you will surely agree with this assessment when you get there. Actually, the beach itself extends into military zones both to the north and to the south, and those areas have been strictly off-limits to public entry since the events of 9/11.

The 1.9-mile stretch in the middle runs from North Beach in the north—or Dog Beach, where pets can roam free and swim—to the south edge of the Coronado Shores high-rise condominium development. In between lies the venerable Hotel del Coronado, affectionately known as the Hotel Del or The Del. Classified as a National Historic Landmark, the hotel first opened its doors in 1888 and was the setting for the shenanigans of the 1959 hit comedy *Some Like It Hot*.

Walking, wading, running, and swimming, not to mention building sand castles, are all popular pursuits here. (Note that pets are allowed only on the northernmost stretch.)

Why is the beach so wide? You'll get a hint when you look at the westward-pointing finger of the Point Loma peninsula. The prevailing California current sweeps south past the point, and some of the flow swirls east and north, depositing sand and sediment along a narrow sandbar called the Silver Strand, just south of Coronado. Plenty of that sand ends up on the shoreline of Coronado itself.

It's especially interesting to walk here during low tide, when the gently shelving wet sand extends far out to sea. Right in front of the hotel, at low tide only, some large rocks intentionally placed there to prevent erosion are exposed. During the lowest tides, some marine life, such as anemones, can be seen clinging to this artificial reef.

THE ROUTE

From wherever you score a parking spot, cross Ocean Boulevard and head across the side beach to the shoreline. A good starting point is the stairway directly across Ocean from Isabella Avenue and leading to the lifeguard tower. Large clean restrooms with showers are available here. (*Note:* At midday, this stretch of dry sand could be fiery hot, so bring at least a pair of flip-flops.) Turn either up-coast or down-coast and make the round-trip. Out-and-back for both segments, combined, totals 3.8 miles. The north turnaround is a fenced barricade at the Naval Air Station North Island boundary. The south turnaround is signed but not fenced at the Naval Amphibious Base just beyond the last high-rise. A military security guard is usually stationed here.

For a really memorable experience, time your visit on a late summer evening when there is a full moon. Plan to be wading north of the Hotel Del at sunset. Can you imagine 70°F water tickling your toes, while at the same time, a big yellow moon launches itself over the fairy-tale turrets of the hotel right in front of you?

TO THE TRAILHEAD

GPS Coordinates: N32° 41.036'   W117° 11.049'

From San Diego, take the toll-free San Diego–Coronado Bridge across San Diego Bay and into Coronado. The westbound lanes become Third Street. After two blocks on Third Street, turn left at the Orange Avenue traffic light. After 1 mile and as you approach the mammoth Victorian-style Hotel del Coronado, turn right on any street beyond 10th Street. They all lead directly or indirectly west to Ocean Boulevard, which runs along the beach. Park on Ocean Boulevard or on any residential street just inland. At this point you'll be roughly in the middle of the publicly accessible stretch of Coronado Beach. This is the area where you will most likely find a parking space.

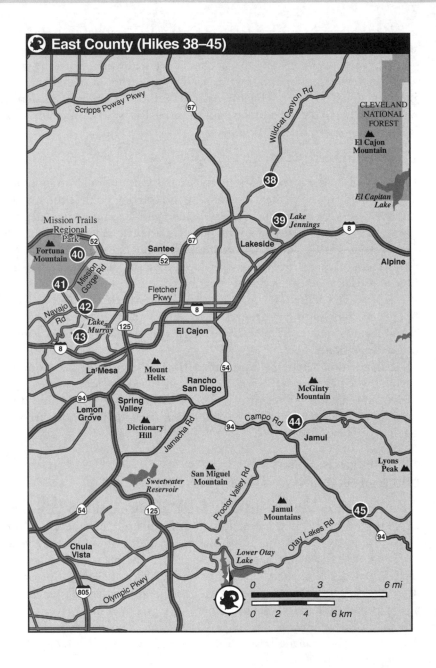

East County (Hikes 38–45)

Scripps Poway Pkwy

67

Wildcat Canyon Rd

CLEVELAND
NATIONAL
FOREST

El Cajon
Mountain

38

El Capitan
Lake

39 Lake
Jennings

8

Mission Trails
Regional
Park

52

Fortuna
Mountain 40

Santee

67

Lakeside

Alpine

52

Mission Gorge Rd

41

Fletcher
Pkwy

Navajo
Rd

42

8

Lake
Murray

125

El Cajon

43

8

La Mesa

Mount
Helix

Rancho
San Diego

54

McGinty
Mountain

94

Lemon
Grove

Spring
Valley

Dictionary
Hill

Jamacha Rd

94 Campo Rd 44

Jamul

Lyons
Peak

Sweetwater
Reservoir

San Miguel
Mountain

Proctor Valley Rd

54

125

Jamul
Mountains

45

94

Chula
Vista

Lower Otay
Lake

Otay Lakes Rd

805

Olympic Pkwy

0   3   6 mi

0   2   4   6 km

EAST COUNTY

What's commonly known among San Diegans as East County spreads inland from the easternmost city limits of San Diego. East County's westside communities—Santee, La Mesa, Lakeside, El Cajon, and Rancho San Diego—are effectively an extension of San Diego's inner-city suburbs.

However, 10–15 miles eastward, only the small communities of Alpine and Jamul, plus scattered rural properties, interrupt the generally wild character of the landscape. Several rocky promontories, such as El Cajon Mountain and Lyons Peak, rise to elevations of 3,000–4,000 feet.

Parks, preserves, and public open-space areas of all sizes are abundant in East County. The flagship Mission Trails Regional Park (more than 7,000 acres following its recent expansion) sits right on the edge of the suburbs, which nearly surround it. Still, it is touted as one of the largest urban parks in the nation. Four of the eight hikes in this section lie inside the borders of Mission Trails Regional Park.

The other four hikes are a little more remote, but all are typically within 30 minutes of downtown San Diego (traffic allowing). Again, as we've seen in earlier sections, these interior hikes are far better experienced in months outside of the July–October hot, dry season.

38 Louis A. Stelzer County Park

Trailhead Location: North of Lakeside

Trail Use: Hiking, running

Distance & Configuration: 2.8-mile loop, including two spurs

Elevation Range: 600'–1,181'

Facilities: Water and restrooms at the trailhead

Highlights: Shade-giving oaks, as well as mountain and valley vistas

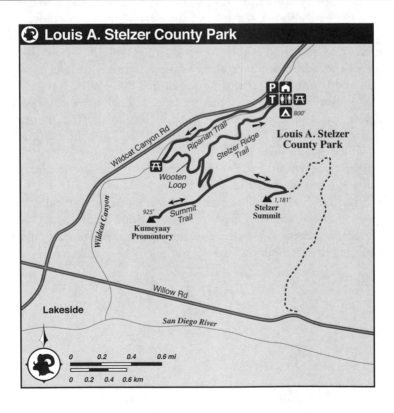

DESCRIPTION

Louis Alexander Stelzer, born in Karlsruhe, Baden-Württemberg, Germany, in 1881, enjoyed a long and successful career as a building contractor and architect in San Diego and Los Angeles. He purchased this property in the 1940s as a weekend retreat he called Shadow Mountain Ranch. When he died at age 91 in 1972, he deeded this property to the county to provide outdoor education and recreation experiences for the children of San Diego. True to Stelzer's wishes, this popular county park features a variety of organized and self-paced activities for kids of all ages, including the Kids in Parks Track Trails program.

The County of San Diego Department of Parks and Recreation operates Louis A. Stelzer County Park, known simply as Stelzer Park, which devotes 420 acres to trails. A core area of campsites, picnic tables, and a small interpretive center nestle in the shady bottom of a steep ravine known as Wildcat Canyon. That area, next to the parking lot, was designed to accommodate persons with disabilities, though all visitors are welcome.

THE ROUTE

From the parking lot, start off by going south, parallel to Wildcat Canyon Road, on the gradually descending Riparian Trail. Before departing, note the posted time for trail closure, which varies seasonally. The trail sticks closely to the stream bottom of Wildcat Canyon. As such, it is semishaded by a stream-hugging canopy of live oaks, some draped with filigrees of wild grape and poison oak vines. The mammoth 2003 Cedar Fire swept through these oaks and into the upper-elevation slopes in this park, but most of the trees have survived more or less intact. Keep an eye out for the tracks of raccoons, coyotes, bobcats, and other "locals" all along this stretch, as well as on the trails above.

After 0.7 mile, the Riparian Trail ends at a secluded picnic site. From there, find and follow the trail marked Wooten Loop, which rises sharply on a slope to the east. After 0.3 mile of climbing, you reach Stelzer Ridge Trail. Hang a right and continue uphill to a wider trail on the ridgeline overlooking Wildcat Canyon.

Once there, for a better view, go 0.3 mile to the right to reach Kumeyaay Promontory. Or go 0.4 mile to the left, up a very steep pitch, toward 1,181-foot Stelzer Summit. At Stelzer Summit, see if you can locate a rock pile atop the nearby hill. There, you will discover a hidden boulder-cave with an opening that overlooks a rural stretch of the San Diego River Valley. When the sea breeze blows up the valley, this becomes surely the

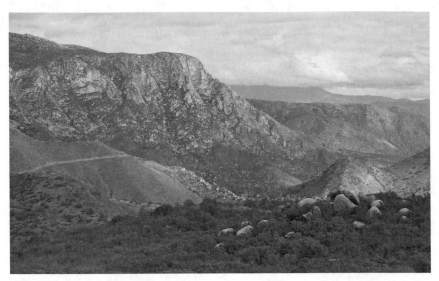
View of El Capitan from Stelzer Ridge

coolest spot within the park. Off in the distance, down the valley, the bedroom communities of Lakeside and Santee spread coastward.

Turning back toward the east while still on Stelzer Summit, pause a few moments to savor the timeless view of El Capitan, El Cajon Mountain's dramatic southern flank. When you are through with the side trips, you may return to the junction of Stelzer Ridge and Wooten Loop. Follow the easily descending Stelzer Ridge Trail back to the park's core area and your starting point.

TO THE TRAILHEAD

GPS Coordinates: N32° 52.993'   W116° 53.819'

From Lakeside, where the CA 67 freeway segment ends at a traffic light, head east on Mapleview Street. After 0.3 mile on Mapleview, turn left (north) on Ashwood Street at the traffic light just beyond the Lakeside Rodeo grounds. Ashwood becomes Wildcat Canyon Road in 1 mile at the four-way stop. From this intersection, proceed 0.8 mile to the signed Stelzer Park entrance on the right.

If coming southbound on CA 67, turn left (east) on Willow Road just north of Lakeside and continue 0.9 mile to the four-way stop at Wildcat Canyon Road, then turn left (north) 0.8 mile to the Stelzer Park entrance. Trailhead parking is available adjacent to the park ranger office. Pay the small fee at a self-service ticket machine just inside the entrance.

39 Lake Jennings

Trailhead Location: Lakeside

Trail Use: Hiking, mountain biking, running

Distance & Configuration: 1.6-mile to 3.3-mile out-and-back with two optional spurs

Elevation Range: 750' at the start to 865'

Facilities: Portable restroom at trailhead; water, restrooms, and bait shop near the lake's entrance

Highlights: Extraordinary springtime color

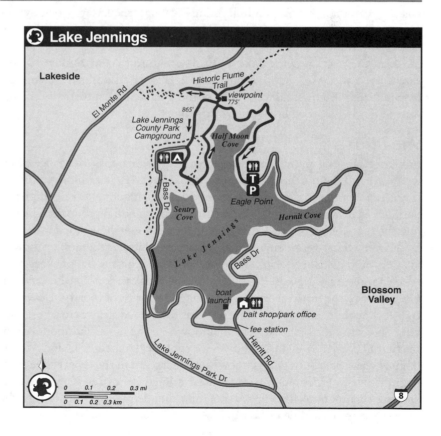

DESCRIPTION

Your impression of Lake Jennings may be strongly colored by the season in which you choose to visit. This is true for many of San Diego County's inland, low-elevation locales. Summer's heat and drought bleach all vibrant color from the vegetation, so that by July—and through the first rainstorms late in the year—the only color you see besides beige and brown is the blue of the sky and of Lake Jennings itself. In most years, though, as is typical for Southern California's Mediterranean climate, February–April brings an almost unbelievable wave of green to the hillsides surrounding the lake. In wetter years the profusion of wildflowers can be astounding.

The Helix Water District owns and administers Lake Jennings, which stores mostly imported water that, when filtered, becomes drinking water for more than a quarter million people in the East County region. For local residents, the lake also serves as a recreational magnet for fishing, boating, camping, hiking, and bicycling—though the latter two activities are not as popular as the first three. But again, the springtime flourish can be dazzling.

Day-use access to the lake is Friday, Saturday, and Sunday. Make sure to stop at the bait shop to purchase tickets for a small per-person fee. Campers may use this trail every day of the week but must turn around just west of Eagle Point, where we start this hike.

THE ROUTE

From the starting point, the nearly level trail (an unpaved service road) wraps around the north shoreline of the lake. The vegetation on the slopes is primarily of the coastal sage scrub variety, which goes almost completely dormant in drought. The plants pack their growth and reproductive phases into the space of a few weeks or months, depending on how much rain falls. By March wildflowers—such as paintbrush, wild hyacinth, monkey flower, lupine, and owl's clover—splash the hillsides with highlights of every hue.

Continue just 0.8 mile to a point on the trail overlooking Half Moon Cove. Notice the broad saddle in the ridge to your right (north). Leave the trail at that point and climb about 50 yards to that saddle, where a gorgeous vista opens to the northeast. You look down on the table-flat floodplain of the San Diego River and in the distance spot rock-ribbed El Cajon Mountain, whose sheer south face is known as El Capitan in these parts due to its resemblance to El Capitan in Yosemite National Park. Retrace your steps, keeping this route to its original 1.6-mile round-trip stroll (including the little segue to the saddle vista).

Or you can continue on toward Lake Jennings's rustic campground on the north shore, where paved Bass Drive resumes; that would turn this route into a 2.6-mile outing featuring a loop if you include the west ridge between the saddle and campground, passing Lake Jennings's high point.

Better yet, continue north beyond the saddle kiosk to intersect and follow a short section of one of San Diego County's newest trails—the Historic Flume Trail. This east-west-trending, nearly level path follows the original course of one of San Diego's earliest civil projects, a remarkable civil engineering achievement of the late 19th century that brought much needed water from the Cuyamaca Mountains to rapidly growing San Diego. Interpretive signs provide historical photos and accounts of celebratory parades and flume rides for San Diegans young and old. Construction of the flume and the dam that impounds Lake Cuyamaca was featured on the cover of the March 15, 1890, issue of *Scientific American* magazine—an early moment of fame for San Diego.

Just below the saddle, a short left spur leads to a barricaded eastern opening of the Monte Tunnel, one of eight that together covered nearly a mile of the original flume route. Although barricaded now, you can still pause here to admire the cut and mortared granite facade. From Monte Tunnel, head 0.2 mile in either direction. Heading east leads to a turnaround at the county's property line. Heading west leads to the top of the switchbacks that take you down to the new Flume Trail trailhead. Both spurs have fine views of El Monte Valley and El Capitan. Return to the saddle to continue toward the campground loop option (3.3 miles total) or back to the Eagle Point trailhead (2.5 miles total).

If you don't mind sharing the road with typically slow-moving vehicles, another option is to circle the lake using Bass Drive—4.6 miles for that entire circuit, not counting the Flume Trail or the campground loop.

TO THE TRAILHEAD
GPS Coordinates: N32° 51.659'   W116° 53.114'

Exit I-8 at Lake Jennings Park Road (Exit 23), just east of El Cajon. Go north about 0.3 mile and bear right onto Harritt Road, following the signs to Lake Jennings. In 0.3 mile, once past the park entrance, stay right, pay the small day-use fee at the bait shop, and continue driving on the winding, paved Bass Drive along the lake's south and east shorelines. After nearly 2 miles, you reach a parking lot where the paved road ends and a hikers' unpaved trail begins.

40 Oak Canyon

Trailhead Location: Mission Gorge, west of Santee

Trail Use: Hiking, dog walking

Distance & Configuration: 3.2-mile out-and-back

Elevation Range: 280'–500'

Facilities: Water and portable toilets at the trailhead

Highlights: A small stream with mini-waterfalls; extravagant springtime vegetation

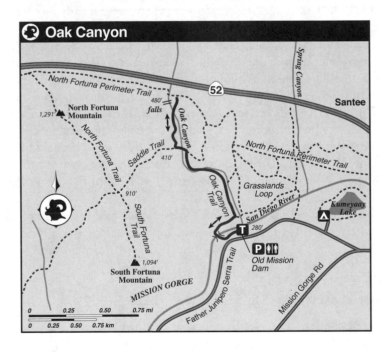

DESCRIPTION

Oak Canyon, a sycamore- and oak-lined ravine that winds north from Mission Gorge's Old Mission Dam, is a perfect place to celebrate the return of spring in San Diego. Heavy rains revive the canyon's intermittent stream and transform the hillside vegetation from dormant brown to festive green.

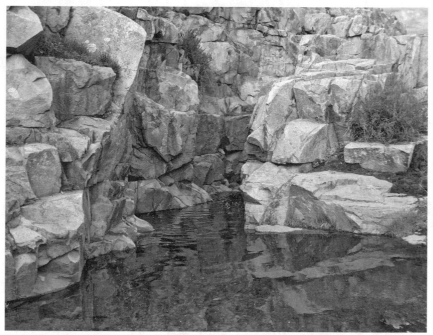

Pool below upper waterfall

By March annual wildflowers pop up amid the tender new blades of grass, blooming ceanothus (wild lilac) and California poppies color the slopes, and the sweet-pungent smell of sage floats on the warm breezes.

THE ROUTE

From the Old Mission Dam parking area, walk west down the wide, smooth path going past various interpretive exhibits and the Old Mission Dam. The dam was built 1803–1816 under the direction of the San Diego Mission and was considered a major engineering feat of its day. A 5-mile-long aqueduct carried water from the dam to the mission at the east end of Mission Valley.

Beyond the exhibits, you cross the often-turbid waters of the San Diego River by way of an iron footbridge. The trail then traverses a sandy stretch of river floodplain and bends right (east) to climb a hillside. After about 100 yards, stay left and descend to the bottom of a shallow ravine— Oak Canyon. In the next 1.2 miles, you'll wend your way upstream along the banks of the trickling creek, passing small cascades and rock-bound pools (in season, of course). Small kids may need a hand in places, and they should be kept well away from the sheer drops where the stream has carved deep into the bedrock. Everyone will enjoy cottontail rabbits scampering through the brush. With some luck, you might flush a covey of quail. Coyotes patrol these spaces, but unless the hour is either very early or very late, you'll likely see no more than tracks and scat.

Avoid any trails that branch right, away from the canyon bottom. At 1.0 mile you will come upon the first of two waterfalls, this one winding over polished granite into a shallow, seasonally filled pool on the left (west) side of the trail. After a refreshing pause here, continue north another 0.2 mile to the path intersection with the Saddle Trail, a dirt access road leading up to Fortuna Saddle and access to both North and South Fortuna Mountains. Turn left (west), follow the road about 100 yards, and go right on a path that continues up Oak Canyon. About 0.3 mile farther, you'll come to a picturesque mini-chasm of water-polished rock with a deep, narrow pool. For a great overview looking back down the canyon, walk another 500 feet north up to the intersection with North Fortuna Perimeter Trail. You could walk farther, but this route ends here, as CA 52 passes over the canyon just ahead on twin high bridges, and off-limits Marine Corps property lies beyond. Return by the same path.

TO THE TRAILHEAD
GPS Coordinates: N32° 50.378'   W117° 2.510'

From the west, exit CA 52 at Mast Boulevard. Turn left (east) on Mast 0.2 mile, then right (south) on West Hills Parkway 0.7 mile to Mission Gorge Road. Turn right (west) and slightly right at Father Junipero Serra Trail. Drive 0.7 mile west on Father Junipero Serra Trail to the Old Mission Dam parking lot on the right. If this lot is full, there is plenty of overflow parking available on the road shoulder outside. You can also access Mission Gorge Road from I-8 in Mission Valley or from northbound CA 125 in Santee.

41 Father Junipero Serra Trail

Trailhead Location: Between San Diego and Santee

Trail Use: Hiking, biking, dog walking, running, skating, night hiking

Distance & Configuration: 4-mile out-and-back; three optional side trails of 0.6–0.8 mile each (5.5 miles when combined)

Elevation Range: 200' at the start to 300' (600' with Climbers Loop option)

Facilities: Water and restrooms at Mission Trails Regional Park Visitor and Interpretive Center and at Old Mission Dam

Highlights: Coastal San Diego County's deepest river gorge

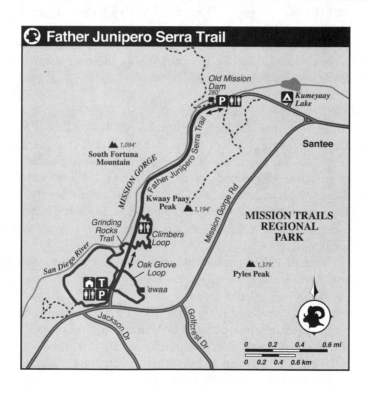

DESCRIPTION

Mission Gorge is arguably the most spectacular topographical feature in the city of San Diego. On both sides of the gorge, walls rise several hundred feet at a nearly 45-degree pitch. From a geological perspective, the gorge was carved out by the "mighty" San Diego River—mighty during Pleistocene times, anyway. The water kept eroding its way through a rising block of tough igneous rock for millions of years. The surrounding granitic peaks—South Fortuna Mountain to the north and Kwaay Paay Peak to the south—were formed more than 100 million years ago from molten rock created deep underground through plate tectonics as the Farallon ocean plate slid beneath the light North American continental plate. As the magma continued to slowly rise, it cooled and crystallized into the granite and was gradually exposed through uplift and erosion to form the cliffs and boulders you see today, all part of the Peninsular Range batholith stretching hundreds of miles between the Santa Ana Mountains and the tip of Baja California. In today's rather dry geologic epoch, there's not as much waterborne excavation going on at the bottom of the gorge, but San Diego's own "old man river" still keeps flowing, mostly lazily, around water-polished granitic rocks and over the roots of gnarled live oaks and rangy sycamores.

THE ROUTE

A single multiuse route threads along the bottom of Mission Gorge today. Actually a paved road called Father Junipero Serra Trail, this route was originally the main, two-lane Mission Gorge Road that connected San Diego's easternmost neighborhoods to Santee. Into the 1960s and '70s, the road still carried secondary car and truck traffic, even after the construction of the four- to six-lane segment of new Mission Gorge Road that bypasses the gorge. Fast-moving semitrucks and recreational cyclists and hikers didn't mix well.

Finally, in the mid-1990s, automotive traffic was nearly eliminated on Father Junipero Serra Trail, and self-propelled travelers at last could feel welcome to use it as a recreational pathway.

The current configuration of Father Junipero Serra Trail is twofold. It features a single, speed bump–studded, eastbound lane that is open during daylight hours for slow-moving automobiles, and it also offers a wide, separate, parallel path for travelers going either direction by foot, bike, or skates. Dog walking is a popular activity as well.

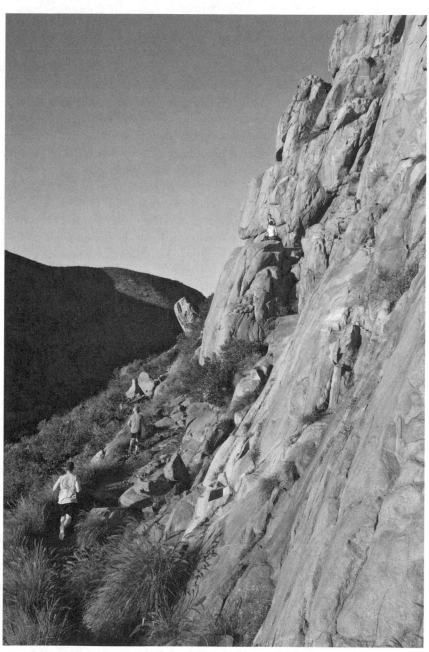

Runners on Climbers Loop

Plentiful free parking is available at either end of the gorge: at the Old Mission Dam historic site off Mission Gorge Road on Santee's west side and at the Mission Trails Regional Park (MTRP) Visitor and Interpretive Center, just east of the Mission Gorge Road and Jackson Drive intersection. Park near the intersection if you want to include a jaunt to the visitor center before or after your hike. Admission is free, and you'll enjoy interpretive displays and commanding views of the gorge.

At the Old Mission Dam side of the trail, you can walk a short distance down to the remnant dam, built in 1816 by American Indian labor secured by the San Diego Mission. The dam, tiny by today's standards, and a 5-mile-long aqueduct facilitated the transfer of water from Mission Gorge to the fertile fields of Mission Valley. The gently rising and falling 2-mile stretch of paved trail in between the visitor center and the Old Mission Dam offers continual vistas of the dramatically soaring walls of the gorge.

Along the north side of Serra Trail the San Diego River slides gently through the cottonwoods and around boulders fallen from the walls of the gorge. Here and there, especially high on the east side, the gorge's granitic bones form an exoskeleton that attracts technical rock climbers from around the region.

While on the paved pathway, keep an eye out for other travelers—from bicyclists zipping around at high speed to kids and pets darting randomly. Also, use caution when exploring any of the side paths so as to avoid any unpleasant encounters with rattlesnakes.

Three optional dirt paths may tempt you to explore off the main paved road. All three begin and end at junctions with Serra Trail and can be incorporated into slightly longer end-to-end hikes.

Oak Grove Loop starts directly east and across Serra Trail from the MTRP Visitor and Interpretive Center. This 0.5-mile loop climbs slightly through open coastal sage scrub, then descends along a seasonal creek beneath a canopy of coast live oak and a stately Engelmann oak, a signature San Diego region species thought to have originated in this area. A replica native Kumeyaay 'ewaa (house) has been constructed near the halfway point.

Grinding Rocks Trail, on the west side of Serra Trail, provides access to the river. Trail junctions include a trailhead directly across from the Oak Grove Loop outlet (0.2 mile from the start) and another at descending stone steps directly across from the Climbers Loop kiosk (0.4 mile from the start). The grinding rocks site features oval and circular depressions in river-polished granite boulders along the south bank of the river. This was a favored area for Kumeyaay women to crush and process locally gathered acorns into a flour that was combined with water and cooked into a mush called *shawee*, a primary food staple. This is a peaceful site beneath the shade of those acorn-producing oaks, accented with birdsong and whispers of the nearby river as it flows past.

Climbers Loop will give you a fitness workout as it climbs steeply on the northwest slopes of Kwaay Paay Peak to the base of the renowned Mission Gorge climbing area. Only 0.8 mile in length, this side path provides exceptional views west toward the visitor center and Mission Valley and an eagle's view out over Mission Gorge and the Serra Trail. On most days, you can watch and hear rock climbers practicing their skills on a variety of challenging routes in the Middle Earth, Underworld, Limbo, or Main Wall areas. As with the other two side trails, Climbers Loop has two entrances from Serra Trail (0.4 mile and 0.6 mile from the start) and can be hiked in either direction.

One way to combine all three options would be to start with Oak Grove Loop. At its outlet cross over Serra Trail to pick up Visitor Center Loop to the right (north) to Grinding Rocks Trail, another right. Signs indicate each of these junctions. Once past Grinding Rocks and up the stone stairs, cross Serra Trail again to the Climbers Loop kiosk for a counterclockwise circuit back to Serra Trail in midcanyon. Turn right again to reach Old Mission Dam, then return for a leisurely stroll back to the visitor center. If the timing and conditions are right, the canyon walls will light up with a marvelous sunset glow.

TO THE TRAILHEAD
GPS Coordinates: N32° 49.200'   W117° 3.423'

The main trailhead, at the MTRP Visitor and Interpretive Center, lies just north of Mission Gorge Road, one long block east of Jackson Drive. From I-8 take the Mission Gorge Road exit (Exit 8), and head 1 mile north on Mission Gorge Road. Turn right to stay on Mission Gorge Road, and continue another 3.2 miles.

From Santee head west on CA 52, and take Exit 13 for Mast Boulevard. Head northeast on Mast Boulevard, and almost immediately turn right on West Hills Parkway. In 0.7 mile turn right on Mission Gorge Road, and go 2.4 miles. The vehicular gate and visitor center parking lot close overnight; street parking is available for after-hours visits.

42 Cowles Mountain

Trailhead Location: San Diego's San Carlos neighborhood, on the city's east side

Trail Use: Hiking, dog walking, running

Distance & Configuration: 3-mile out-and-back

Elevation Range: 660' at the trailhead to 1,591' at the top

Facilities: Water and restrooms at the trailhead; snack shop and convenience store across the street

Highlights: Simply the most comprehensive vista any peak in San Diego can offer

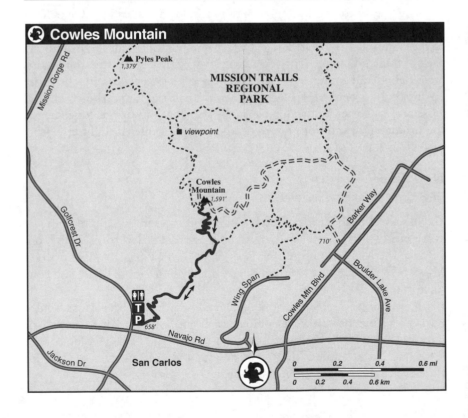

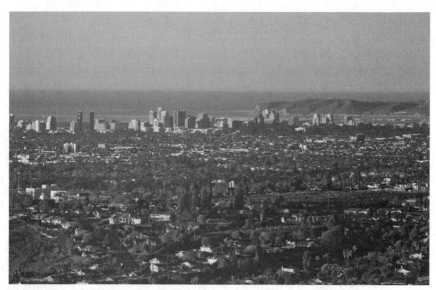

Early morning trail view of downtown San Diego and Point Loma

DESCRIPTION

For good reason, this switchback trail is the most heavily trafficked hiking route in all of San Diego County. The route ascends the sunny south side of Cowles Mountain to the summit—at 1,591 feet, it is the highest point within San Diego's city limits and Mission Trails Regional Park (MTRP). At more than 7,000 acres, MTRP is one of the largest urban parks in the nation.

Cowles Mountain is named for a pioneering rancher George A. Cowles (pronounced "coals"), who settled just east of here in 1877. His two ranches were called Woodside and Magnolia. Cowles was known around the country for his grapes, olives, wheat, and potatoes grown and shipped from here. The area around Woodside Ranch was originally called Cowlestown. In 1887 George passed away, and in 1890 his widow, Jennie, married his partner, Milton Santee, a real estate developer. In 1893 Cowlestown was renamed Santee, as it remains today.

Because of the low-growing coastal sage scrub vegetation, you and your fellow hikers will enjoy unobstructed views nearly the entire way up. At first, nearby features such as Lake Murray command your attention. Then far-off locales—Mexico, downtown San Diego, and the Pacific Ocean—come into view.

The trail was cut on mostly decomposed granite, so it is quite susceptible to erosion wherever the slope gets steep. Please don't shortcut the switchbacks, tempting as it may be on the way up or down, as this aggravates the erosion problem. Wear sturdy shoes, as jutting rocks and wicked little ruts sometimes punctuate the trail surface. Also, consider not doing this climb when the weather is hot and sunny. It's easy to become dehydrated and woozy, and you'll need all of your faculties to negotiate the rough patches on the way down. Starting the climb early to catch the sunrise is a great way to begin your day—see and hear San Diego come to life from this lofty perch. Sunsets can be equally spectacular to watch from the summit. Carry along plenty of drinking water, of course, and a headlamp or flashlight for those predawn ascents or evening twilight returns.

THE ROUTE

From the trailhead, make your way up the zigzagging and occasionally heavily eroded trail, which climbs relentlessly through low-growing sage scrub and chaparral. By 0.7 mile, you're passing scattered outcrops of rounded granitic rock, which add to the aesthetic pleasure of the widening panorama. At a spot 0.9 mile beyond your starting point, the main trail bends sharply left.

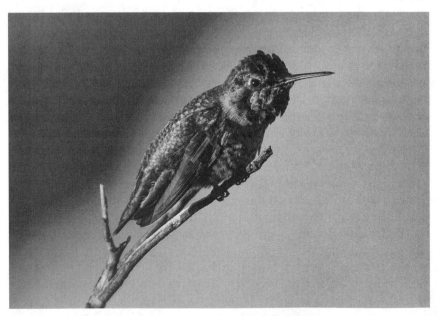

Anna's hummingbird

Beyond the bend, a little farther upslope at 1 mile from the start, a through-trail branches right, heading eastward toward Barker Way at the mountain's east base. Stay left and continue up the mountainside on the series of long switchback segments leading to the rocky summit of the mountain. A concrete monument marks the high point, and two large interpretive panels stand nearby, with the names and directions of major features visible along the horizon.

A blocky building bristling with microwave dishes obstructs the northward view somewhat, but otherwise the panorama is complete. With binoculars and a street map, you may be lulled into spending a lot of time identifying features on the urban landscape. In the rift between the coastal terrace to the west, there's a good view of Mission Valley and the tangle of freeways that pass over and through it. Southwest, the high-rise buildings of downtown San Diego stand against Point Loma, Coronado, and San Diego Bay. Lake Murray shimmers to the south, and sprawling Tijuana, Mexico, rolls across the mesas and ravines on the southern horizon. The chain of Santee Lakes contrasts darkly with pale hills to the north. In all directions, you look down on the abodes of many of the more than 3 million people who live within a 35-mile radius of where you stand.

On clear winter days, the view expands to include most of the higher peaks of San Diego County. Southward into Baja, you can see the flat-topped Table Mountain beyond Tijuana and the Coronado Islands off-shore. During absolutely crystalline weather, look for the profiles of Santa Catalina and San Clemente Islands, to the northwest and west respectively.

After you've gaped sufficiently at the surrounding landscape, or perhaps finished your trailside snack or lunch, turn around and return exactly as you came. But be especially cautious on the way down. Remember those steep and eroded sections of trail that you covered on the way up? Observe such rough areas and descend accordingly. As noted in the Introduction, this is a very popular trail but arguably presents the most challenging descent among all 50 routes in this book.

TO THE TRAILHEAD
GPS Coordinates: N32° 48.286'   W117° 2.243'

Exit I-8 at College Avenue (Exit 10), and go north 1.3 miles. Turn right on Navajo Road, and continue 2 miles east to the Cowles Mountain Trailhead on the northeast corner of Navajo Road and Golfcrest Drive. A small parking lot fills early, but street parking is available along Golfcrest.

43 Lake Murray

Trailhead Location: La Mesa, just east of San Diego

Trail Use: Hiking, dog walking, running, biking, skating, night hiking

Distance & Configuration: 6.2-mile out-and-back

Elevation Range: About 550' throughout

Facilities: Water, restrooms, and small concession stand at the start; pit toilets along the route; water at a drinking fountain next to some baseball fields at Lake Murray Community Park on the north shore

Highlights: Fresh breezes and sparkling lake views all along the route; superb bird-watching opportunities

DESCRIPTION

Lake Murray is eastern San Diego's most pleasant and most popular place to gulp some fresh air just about any time of year. Earlier or later on most days, hundreds of runners, speed walkers, skaters, and cyclists dodge each other on the lake's perimeter service road (closed to automobiles) that extends along about four-fifths of the lake's shoreline. Thus, the road's end, about 3 miles out from the start, makes this route an out-and-back rather than a pleasing lake loop.

Lake Murray also provides an excellent bird-watching opportunity. Be sure to bring binoculars to visually capture the lake's mix of aquatic fowl (ducks, coots, white pelicans, great blue herons, nesting ospreys, and much more) and also the freewheeling large birds (hawks, ravens, and vultures) in the sky overhead.

THE ROUTE

From the easternmost parking area beyond the lake entrance, start your walk at the perimeter road, which is gated to block vehicles. Eucalyptus and jacaranda trees spread shade over the road along the way, but mostly this route is open to the warm sun; thus hikers and runners much prefer the early morning and late afternoon hours. (A contingent of early risers from the adjacent neighborhood often walks the lake route as early as 5 a.m.)

After swinging around four fingerlike arms of the lake, the publicly accessible part of the road comes to an end at a formidable fence just shy

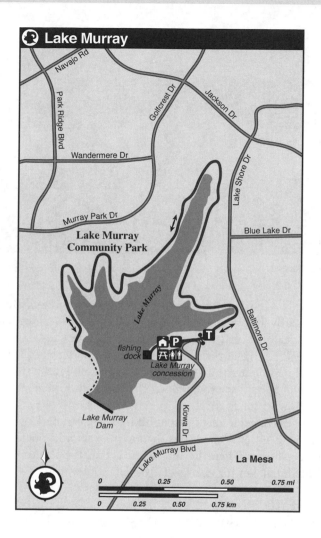

Lake Murray

Navajo Rd

Park Ridge Blvd

Golfcrest Dr

Jackson Dr

Wandermere Dr

Lake Shore Dr

Murray Park Dr

**Lake Murray
Community Park**

Blue Lake Dr

Lake Murray

Baltimore Dr

fishing
dock

P

T

Lake Murray
concession

Lake Murray
Dam

Kiowa Dr

Lake Murray Blvd

La Mesa

| 0 | 0.25 | 0.50 | 0.75 mi |
| 0 | 0.25 | 0.50 | 0.75 km |

of the west abutment of the Lake Murray Dam. There's no passage across the narrow concrete dam ahead, which was completed in 1919, so you must turn back and return from there. Make sure to touch the bull's-eye at the turnaround.

You'll likely enjoy this far-end section of the perimeter road best. A wild, rocky, scruffy hillside rises to the west, housing a cohort of coyotes, whose howls announce their presence after dark. To the east spreads the sometimes glassy, sometimes wind-rippled surface of the lake, flecked with rowboats

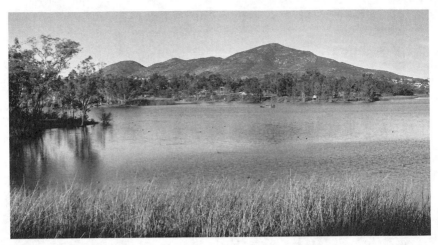

Lake Murray and Cowles Mountain

and small fishing craft. Cowles Mountain accents the east horizon. Birds find this side particularly attractive, so make sure to point your binoculars toward the shoreline reeds, shrubs, and overhanging tree branches.

On your way back from the turnaround point, you may consider following any of several paralleling trails that diverge from and later return to the paved main road. You will see them along the shoreline and along the slopes above the perimeter road.

Another activity to consider here is night hiking. You can park outside the entrance gate, walk in, and enjoy the shadowy sights and nocturnal sounds along the lakeshore. When the full moon is out, the shimmering surface of Lake Murray makes for an especially memorable stroll.

TO THE TRAILHEAD

GPS Coordinates: N32º 47.080'   W117º 02.535'

From I-8 in La Mesa, take the Lake Murray Boulevard exit (Exit 11). Drive 0.5 mile north to Kiowa Drive, and turn left (north). Kiowa dead-ends at the Lake Murray gate, which is open during daylight hours. Parking is free in several lots inside.

44 McGinty Mountain

Trailhead Location: East of Jamul in southern San Diego County

Trail Use: Hiking, dog walking, running, mountain biking

Distance & Configuration: 4.6-mile out-and-back

Elevation Range: 880'–2,183'

Facilities: None at the trailhead; commercial facilities in Jamul, 1 mile southwest

Highlights: Superb views along route and from summit, fragrant coastal sage scrub, historic mining prospects

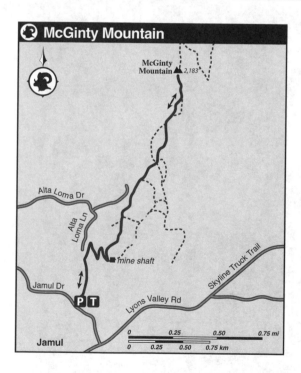

DESCRIPTION

Rising like a scruffy whaleback above a sea of luxury homes, McGinty Mountain hosts a rich but circumspect treasure of botanical oddities.

Several rare and endangered plant species make their home here on soils derived from a relatively uncommon form of bedrock called gabbro. These soils are low in mineral elements normally essential to plants and high in toxic elements like iron and heavy metals, an environment requiring unique adaptations for these specialists to survive and thrive. More than half of California's remaining specimens of Dehesa nolina cling to the mountain's rocky spine. The endemic San Diego thornmint, its habitat reduced by 90% due to urbanization over the last century, survives here, as does San Miguel

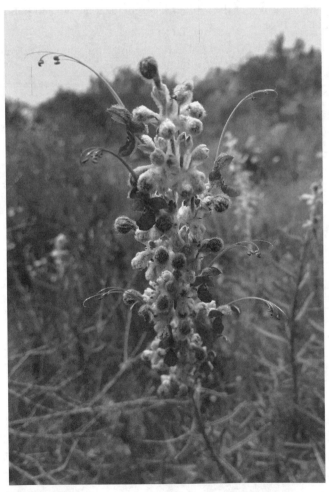

Woolly bluecurls

savory, Parry's tetracoccus, and San Diego (Gander's) butterweed. Some of these plants are believed to be relict species, once common but now almost squeezed out of existence by gradual climate changes occurring over the past 10,000 years or more.

The Nature Conservancy acquired most of the McGinty land from the Bureau of Land Management (BLM) in 1983, when the BLM sought to dispose of isolated lands it could not properly manage. Additional purchases of private land increased the McGinty Mountain Ecological Reserve's size and made it possible to construct a public access trail. Today, McGinty Mountain is within an extensive ecological reserve comanaged by The Nature Conservancy, the California Department of Fish and Wildlife, and the U.S. Fish and Wildlife Service as part of the San Diego National Wildlife Refuge.

THE ROUTE

From the reserve entrance on Jamul Drive, follow the wide trail north, alongside a shallow draw. After 0.33 mile, branch right on a switchback trail that quickly rises to McGinty Mountain's long south ridge. Trained eyes might pick out some of the rarer plants, but mostly you'll notice that the typical sage scrub and chaparral vegetation, attractively green and very aromatic, are moistened by winter rains. Look for the somewhat unusual coast spice bush (a member of the citrus family) and chaparral yucca, also known as Our Lord's candle, whose tall flower stalks bear white blossom clusters in early spring.

The trail tops out at a T 0.75 mile from the switchback section. Just to your right at 200 feet is an opening to one of several prospects and mine shafts located on the flanks of McGinty Mountain. Little is known about McGinty aside from the fact that he owned these small mines, which produced material used in the manufacture of ceramic products, including porcelain. McGinty aplite (a light granite) was shipped throughout the United States and to Great Britain. Though this low-ceilinged shaft may look inviting, mines are intrinsically dangerous places, so for your safety, please don't enter.

Turn back toward the switchback junction and continue ascending more gradually toward the first ridgetop. At 1.0 mile, you meet an old dirt road on top of the ridge. Turn left (north) to set a course for McGinty Mountain's 2,183-foot rounded summit, another 1.3 miles away. You'll be returning on the same route, so take note of any intersecting roads that might cause confusion on your way back. In a few places, this road is very steep and rocky.

Clumps of Dehesa nolina, looking somewhat like poor cousins of the common yuccas, dot the ridgeline. They can be identified by their diminutive stature and fibrous, pale-green, ribbonlike leaves. As you climb the ridge, the fragrance of Cleveland sage—probably the most pleasantly aromatic plant in the county—is almost overpowering, especially in springtime.

The panoramic view expands as you get higher, easily encompassing most of the border-region peaks from Tecate Peak to San Miguel Mountain. In the upper section, additional mining shafts are visible just across the canyon to the west. To the east, triangular, chaparral-cloaked Sycuan Peak rises to 2,801 feet, more than 600 feet higher than McGinty Mountain, with an equally commanding view. Off to the west, beyond Mount Helix and Cowles Mountain, you can sometimes spot the ocean—dark blue or glistening with sun glare depending on the time of day.

After taking in the grand sights atop McGinty's rock-strewn summit, return by the same route.

TO THE TRAILHEAD

GPS Coordinates: N32° 43.770'   W116° 52.345'

From San Diego, take CA 94 east. Continue beyond where the freeway ends, and at the third traffic light (Campo Road), turn right to remain on CA 94. Continue 4.5 miles to the rural community of Jamul. Turn left (east) on Lyons Valley Road, and go 0.75 mile, then turn left (north) on Jamul Drive. A small dirt parking lot with an information kiosk is 0.4 mile ahead on the right.

45 Hollenbeck Canyon

Trailhead Location: East of Jamul in southern San Diego County

Trail Use: Hiking, dog walking, running, mountain biking, horseback riding

Distance & Configuration: 4.4-mile out-and-back or 5.6-mile balloon

Elevation Range: 770'–1,320'

Facilities: Portable restroom but no water at the trailhead; commercial facilities in Jamul, 4 miles west

Highlights: Stately oaks, stunning springtime-green vegetation and wildflowers, and seasonal waterfall

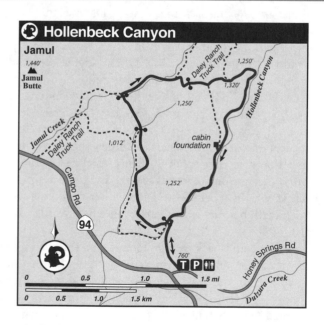

DESCRIPTION

Formerly part of a working ranch, Hollenbeck Canyon is now a California Department of Fish and Game wildlife area covering more than 6,000 acres. While primarily serving as protected habitat for birds, animals, and native vegetation, portions are open to all types of nonmotorized travel, plus a bit of seasonal bird hunting.

Like many low-elevation inland locales in San Diego County, Hollenbeck Canyon has a Jekyll and Hyde personality, sunblasted and desolate for the most part in summer and gloriously green—almost lush—in the winter and early spring, when splashes of wildflower color may be found all along this hike. This dichotomy is due purely to the prevailing Mediterranean climate of winter-wet, summer-dry. Down along the canyon bottom itself, however, water (either on the surface or underground during the dry seasons) nourishes shade-giving trees. And the shrubby and grassy hillside vegetation that goes dormant during droughts comes alive with frenzied growth in the weeks following the winter rains. Those rains replenish a seasonal creek with cascades and a waterfall viewable from the upper canyon trail. For this reason, January–April is typically the best time to hike here.

THE ROUTE

There are a few options: an out-and-back to a T with Daley Ranch Truck Trail (4.4 miles round-trip) or a loop of 5.6–6.4 miles, each of which start from the trailhead parking area. A 0.3-mile passage across an often-parched, treeless meadow hardly prepares you for the idyllic scene soon to come. You pass a yellow-topped post marking the route of the historic California Riding and Hiking Trail and descend gently into shallow Hollenbeck Canyon. At this point, the canyon is lined by an agreeable collection of massive coast live oaks and leafy California sycamores. One of the first oaks in sight is a grizzled, misshapen specimen that not only has survived past fires but that also rises some 50 feet into the sky. The trail soon curves left to cross the canyon's seasonal stream and joins a dirt road. For the out-and-back stay right (north)—and remember this juncture on your way back when you will be tracing this same route backward. For the loop, turn left (south).

Continuing with the out-and-back, you go alongside a thin green strip of willow trees, mule fat shrubs, and other riparian vegetation, with a stray Engelmann oak or two joining the coast live oaks and sycamores. Engelmanns, with their smooth grayish-green leaves and elongated acorns, are thought to have originated in the San Diego region, so they are truly native. The slopes of the canyon, clothed in a veneer of sage scrub vegetation, gradually close in tighter. From this vantage, no sign of civilization save the road you walk on is apparent. The wind whispers in fluttering leaves.

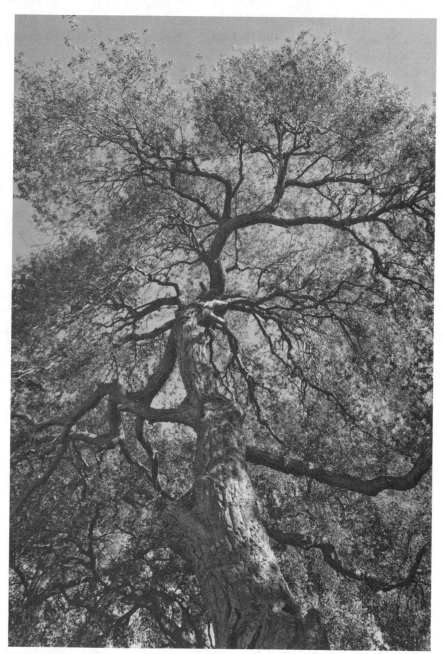

Towering oak

At 1.3 miles from the start (if taking the out-and-back), a side path goes left about 50 yards to the foundation remains of a cabin. Returning to the main route, and soon afterward, a side trail diverges to the right from the wider path that climbs along a broad ridge. Take the more interesting of the two—the path to the right. It threads the eroded west wall of the narrowing gorge ahead. At 2.0 miles, a short section of stonework supports the trail as it passes above the narrows of Hollenbeck Canyon, where floodwaters tumbling down from upstream Lyons Valley have cut a nearly vertical trench in the bedrock. Off in the distance, eastward, soars the rocky summit of Lyons Peak. In another 0.2 mile you reach a T with the Daley Ranch Truck Trail and logical end to the out-and-back option; turn around here and retrace the same 2.2 miles back to the trailhead, staying left at each junction.

One of several loops can be traveled either clockwise or counterclockwise. A clockwise route is described here as it descends rather than climbs the steepest section of road and incorporates two lesser-traveled singletrack sections. Starting from the trailhead, hike north to the first stream crossing near the 0.5-mile post. Turn left (south). In a little over 100 yards, a singletrack branches to the right. Turn here, follow the path until it intersects

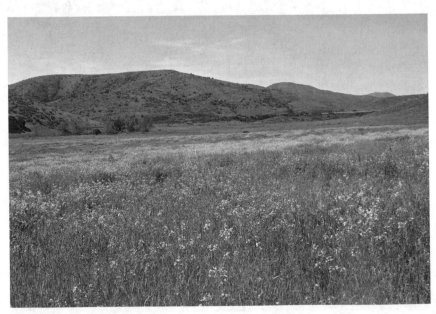

Flowers along the west loop

one of the old ranch roads, and climb gradually into a long valley to merge with another ranch road (wooden post marked 4.6-MILE SHORTCUT).

Just ahead, another singletrack angles off to the right through fields of tall grasses and, in springtime, delightful California poppies, fiddle-necks, and other wildflowers. Pass through the picturesque remnant of an old ranch gate and keep straight (north), heading across a shallow ravine, then up a section of rutted road to a saddle. This is a good spot to survey where you have been and where you are going. Descend to a peaceful, shady grove of oaks, cross usually dry Jamul Creek, and turn right (east), following Daley Ranch Truck Trail parallel to a dilapidated barbwire fence on your right. Continue east on the road 0.5 mile past a branching junction on the left (north) that leads to a spring and water tank in Jamul Creek canyon.

In another 0.5 mile, you pass a T junction on your right (south), where a wooden post is marked 4.2 MILES. Continue straight, though, up another 0.25 mile to a sharp hairpin turn at 1,320 feet, the high point of the loop hike. Pause a moment along this section to take in the panoramic view south out over rolling hills all the way to Otay Mountain, which dominates the horizon. Depart the truck trail here to descend a dirt road steeply downward to the east for 0.25 mile just before reaching a small seasonal creek. Take the trail to the right (south). This is the turnaround point described earlier for the out-and-back option. Return to the trailhead in reverse order of the earlier trail description.

TO THE TRAILHEAD

GPS Coordinates: N32° 40.243'   W116° 49.390'

From San Diego, take CA 94 east. Continue beyond where the freeway ends, and at the third traffic light (Campo Road), turn right to remain on CA 94. Continue 5 miles to the rural community of Jamul, and go an additional 4 miles on CA 94 to Honey Springs Road, on the left. Make a left, go 0.1 mile, and enter the large parking lot to the left, which serves as the Hollenbeck Canyon Trailhead and equestrian staging area.

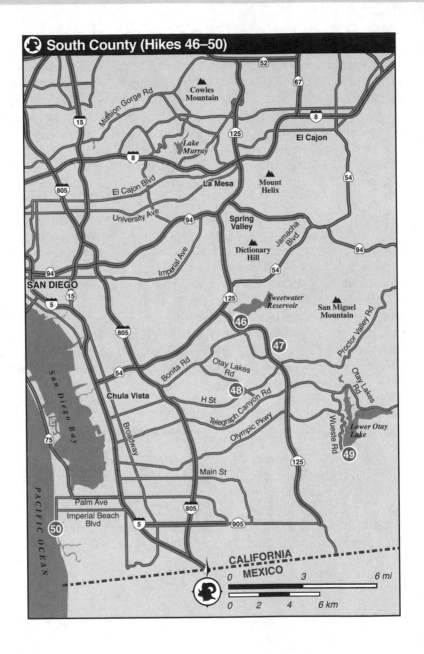

South County (Hikes 46–50)

52

67

Cowles
Mountain

15

8

El Cajon

Mission Gorge Rd

Lake
Murray

125

8

805

El Cajon Blvd

La Mesa

Mount
Helix

54

University Ave

94

Spring
Valley

94

Imperial Ave

Dictionary
Hill

Jamacha
Blvd

54

SAN DIEGO

15

5

125

Sweetwater
Reservoir

San Miguel
Mountain

Proctor Valley Rd

805

46

47

54

Bonita Rd

Otay Lakes
Rd

Otay Lakes
Rd

Chula Vista

H St

48

Telegraph Canyon Rd

Broadway

Olympic Pkwy

Wueste Rd

Lower Otay
Lake

49

75

Main St

125

San Diego Bay

Palm Ave

Imperial Beach
Blvd

805

5

905

50

PACIFIC OCEAN

CALIFORNIA

MEXICO

0   3   6 mi

0   2   4   6 km

SOUTH COUNTY

South County, or the South Bay region as it is often called, spreads inland some 10 miles from the shores of South San Diego Bay. Chock-full of housing and industrial developments near the bay shore, the region gradually assumes a suburban and, finally, a semirural character as you travel east. Beyond the housing developments, rounded peaks and mountain ranges rise from rolling hills and broad valleys. Much of this relatively empty zone is filling up with residences accommodating much of San Diego County's future population growth.

The five hikes in this section have been chosen for ease of access. All feature well-defined trailheads. Parking (with the possible exclusion of Hike 50, Imperial Beach, in the summer) is not a problem. Warm and dry midsummer days on routes such as Hike 46, the Sweetwater Trail, and Hike 47, Mother Miguel Mountain, warrant an early start or an extralarge water bottle. The other three South County hikes are short or easy and carefree.

46 Sweetwater Trail

Trailhead Location: Bonita

Trail Use: Hiking, dog walking, running, mountain biking, horseback riding

Distance & Configuration: 4.6-mile out-and-back

Elevation Range: 230' to 480' at the viewpoint

Facilities: Water and restrooms at the start

Highlights: Panoramic views of South San Diego County's mountain and foothill communities

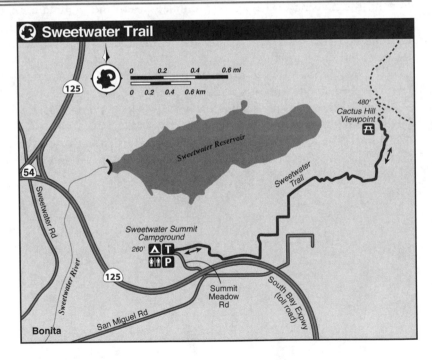

DESCRIPTION

San Diego's South Bay region—the coastal plain and foothills inland from South San Diego Bay—mixes up square miles' worth of recently built housing tracts with pristine meadows and mountain slopes, albeit treeless ones. You can still find wide-open spaces where wild oats and foxtails chafe in the afternoon breeze, the spicy aroma of sage scents the air, hawks glide overhead, and coyotes and other small animals flourish.

One such space surrounds Sweetwater Reservoir in the semirural community of Bonita. Long before any significant modern settlement of the area, the Sweetwater Dam was built to impound the rather meager flow of runoff from mountains to the east and dole it out to agricultural lands during the summer dry season. At the time of its completion in 1888, the dam was higher than any other dam of its kind in the United States. Today, the dam and reservoir are merely bantam class, but they're a lovely addition to the landscape nonetheless.

Sensuously rounded hills—dotted with sage, pepper trees, and rare coastal varieties of cholla and barrel cactus—spread to the south and east of Sweetwater Reservoir, adjacent to the more than 11,000 acres of San Diego National Wildlife Refuge. Within the refuge but not accessible are vernal pools, home to federally endangered San Diego fairy shrimp and threatened native bird species, including coastal California gnatcatchers. Running-shoe footprints overlap the linear marks of mountain bike tires, the inverted U impressions of horseshoes, and an occasional baby hand–shaped raccoon track on the Sweetwater Trail that skirts the shore of the reservoir.

THE ROUTE

You pick up the best section of the Sweetwater Trail at the north end of Sweetwater Summit Campground. Head east, first passing a fishing access area for the reservoir and then traversing near-flat grassland. It's hot in the middle of the day, perhaps, but it's pleasant in early morning or late afternoon.

After about 1 mile, the trail veers sharply right and begins a series of relentless and rather severe ups and downs. You're aiming for the flat top of a prominent knoll ahead—Cactus Hill Viewpoint—where you'll find a picnic table under a shade ramada with a commanding view of the lake and much of the South Bay area. In the opposite direction rises the massive, triangular bulk of San Miguel Mountain, its summit bewhiskered by several spiky radio and TV broadcast antennas.

This fine view spot, 2.4 miles into the hike, is a good place to turn around. It is the termination point for this 4.8-mile route.

If you want to keep going, some additional 2 miles of hiking will get you to the foot of San Miguel Mountain. Beyond that, it is possible to follow trails and dirt paths paralleling the Sweetwater River all the way to CA 94 at Rancho San Diego.

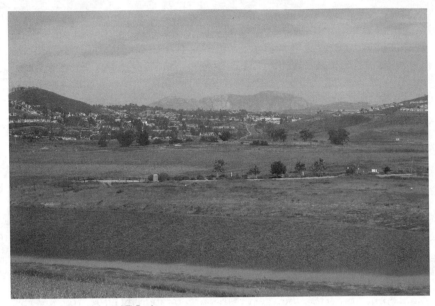

Sweetwater Reservoir and El Capitan

TO THE TRAILHEAD
GPS Coordinates: N32° 41.021'   W117° 0.105'

Exit I-805 at Bonita Road (Exit 7C) and go east about 4 miles. Keep going straight on San Miguel Road at the intersection where Bonita Road swings abruptly north and crosses the Sweetwater River. After 1-plus mile on San Miguel Road, turn left on Summit Meadow Road, which leads to the north end of Sweetwater Summit Campground, the starting point for the hike. (*Note:* There is no access to San Miguel Road from the CA 125 toll road that passes over it.)

47 Mother Miguel Mountain

Trailhead Location: Chula Vista

Trail Use: Hiking, mountain biking, leashed-dog walking

Distance & Configuration: 5-mile out-and-back

Elevation Range: 680' at the start to 1,509' at the summit

Facilities: Parking, water, and restrooms at nearby Mount San Miguel Community Park

Highlights: Panoramic views, wildlife refuge, native plants, endangered butterfly

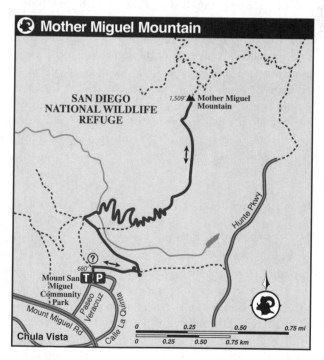

DESCRIPTION

Featuring some of the very best views of sprawling South County, reliable ocean breezes, and exceptional native habitats for springtime wildflowers and year-round native fauna, including several rare or endangered species,

Mother Miguel Mountain well deserves the accolades it gets from knowledgeable locals. Situated just west of taller San Miguel Mountain (not open to the public) and to the southeast of Sweetwater Reservoir, Mother Miguel is a popular destination for hikers and mountain bikers and anyone looking for a great outdoor workout. Think StairMaster on steroids!

Our route crosses San Diego Gas & Electric property and the San Diego National Wildlife Refuge (open sunrise–sunset). The refuge, managed by the U.S. Fish & Wildlife Service, is home to the endangered Quino checkerspot butterfly, recently reintroduced from pupae by volunteers and biologists from San Diego Zoo, U.S. Fish & Wildlife Service, San Diego State University, and the Conservation Biology Institute. Wildlife you might encounter include desert cottontails, coyotes, bobcats, mule deer, a host of smaller mammals, and a variety of resident and migrating birds. Roadrunners are often sighted here carrying recently captured prey, typically lizards or field mice or voles. The San Diego cactus wren, a state-designated species of special concern, also calls the refuge home, in one of the few remaining coastal sage scrub habitats that is suitable for their breeding success and protected from residential development. Please stay on the trail while within the refuge to help avoid negatively impacting Mother Miguel's residents.

At the 1,509-foot summit stands a large rock pile visible for miles. The original Rockhouse Trail led to a namesake feature with low enclosed walls near the high point. Although it is possible to continue beyond, the rock pile serves as our turnaround point for this hike.

THE ROUTE

Our route starts from the north end of Paseo Veracruz. A short 150 feet ahead is a small trailhead kiosk with a satellite map showing the recommended hiking path. Rather than continuing straight ahead at this junction, the currently authorized trail takes a turn to the right (east) and continues up the broad, relatively new city trail passing behind neighborhood backyards for 0.25 mile to a white concrete highway barricade on your left. Cross to the north side of the barricade and walk northeast a few more yards, then turn sharply left and follow a descending dirt road to the northwest that parallels a ravine on your right. In another 0.4 mile you reach a T-junction with the original trail. Turn right and descend into and across a seasonal creek. You are soon in the San Diego National Wildlife Refuge. If visiting in the spring, especially following a wet winter season, the wildflowers can be extraordinary in numbers and variety. Examples

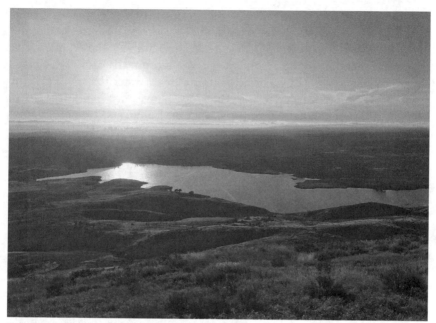

Coastal fog and sun from the summit of Mount Miguel

include our own San Diego County sunflower, splendid mariposa lily, checkerbloom, bush mallow, and, if you look closely, Nuttall's snapdragon.

After crossing the creekbed, follow the winding switchback trail up the southwest ridge of Mother Miguel. There are plans to rebuild the trail with a more habitat-friendly route that avoids the steep, heavily trafficked, and deeply eroded fall line route. That project, funded in part by the San Diego Association of Governments as a grant to the refuge and by the San Diego Mountain Biking Association, will also install directional signs to help guide traffic away from impacted areas and may be complete by the time you read this.

In this eco-friendly spirit and until the new path is constructed, our route stays on the original switchbacks up to the first plateau, where the main route gains its first views of nearby San Miguel Mountain to the northeast, rocky Lyons Peak off to the east, and sprawling Otay Mountain to the southeast. From here the expanse of South Bay unfolds below you and extends southward into Tijuana and the mountains of coastal Baja California. Late afternoon lighting on these prominent local summits can be spectacular.

The remainder of our hike to the summit rock pile follows a wide established route. Once on top, soak in the cool, onshore breeze, sometimes an impressively strong wind in late afternoon, and the panoramic views in every direction. To the northeast rise the steep walls of East County's signature El Capitan (El Cajon Mountain). Sweetwater Reservoir and the route of Hike 46 lies below you to the west. Downtown San Diego's skyline, the prominent whaleback profile of Point Loma, and the shimmering Pacific Ocean grace the horizon.

Most of the rock house walls have been dismantled over time to create a variety of new formations, including a large skyward-facing peace sign. Please avoid moving rocks or contributing to further degradation of the refuge's sensitive habitat.

Return by the same path, including following the switchbacks where available. Check with the refuge for updates on the new trail's status.

TO THE TRAILHEAD

GPS Coordinates: N32° 40.320'   W116° 58.328'

Exit I-805 at Bonita Road (Exit 7C) and go east 3.5 miles. Continue straight on San Miguel Road 0.9 mile and turn right (south) on Proctor Valley Road. In 0.5 mile turn left (east) on San Miguel Ranch Road. Continue 1.4 miles on San Miguel Ranch Road, which becomes Mount Miguel Road. Turn left (north) on Paseo Veracruz and continue 0.2 mile to street parking near the trailhead. The entrance to facilities at Mount San Miguel Community Park is on the left just south of the trailhead.

48 Rice Canyon

Trailhead Location: Chula Vista

Trail Use: Hiking, dog walking, mountain biking, running

Distance & Configuration: 3.6-mile out-and-back

Elevation Range: 350' at the trailhead; 200' at the turnaround point

Facilities: Water and public restrooms at Discovery Park, near the trailhead

Highlights: Easy strolling along a still-natural patch of canyon landscape

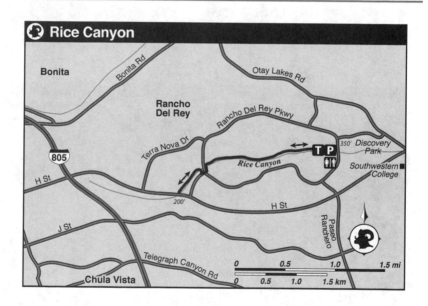

DESCRIPTION

On the scrub-covered slopes of Rice Canyon, hardy coast cholla cacti raise their asymmetric arms in what seems like a gesture of defiance against the surrounding phalanxes of cookie-cutter, pseudo Spanish–style homes. Native California sunflowers and San Diego County sunflowers paint the slopes with splashes of bright yellow. What remains of the formerly obscure and totally rural Rice Canyon has been incorporated into the city of Chula

Vista's Rice Canyon Open Space Preserve. A fine, wide trail follows it nearly 2 miles, down to as far as H Street, 1 mile east of I-805.

Spring is by far the best time to enjoy the sights and fragrances of the canyon's plant life, most of which is classified as native riparian and coastal sage scrub. The handy "Plant Guide to Rice Canyon" is available at the trailhead kiosk or from the City of Chula Vista website (chulavistaca.gov). This color brochure features photos and descriptions of 36 different species of native plants found here. The largest bushes in sight along the trail and on the canyon slopes are lemonade berry shrubs. American Indians once used the shrubs' sticky fruit to prepare a beverage similar to lemonade.

The canyon is also home to a variety of local four-legged critters, typically more active after dark, including coyotes, bobcats, and raccoons. See if you can identify their tracks, especially visible after rain.

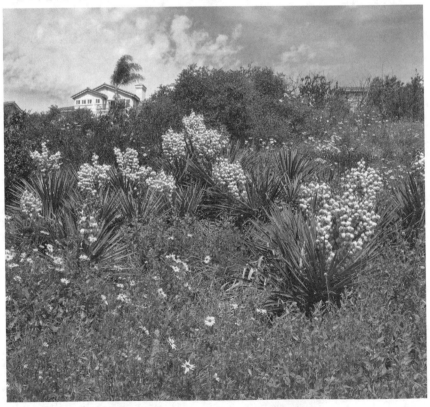

California sunflowers, yucca blossoms, and coast cholla

THE ROUTE

From the sidewalk on the west side of Rancho Del Rey Parkway, across from Discovery Park, start heading west on the wide Rice Canyon Trail. A modernistic trailhead sculpture points to the North Star. Brown and yellow posts signal that this is also a remnant section of the California Riding and Hiking Trail, originally envisioned in 1945 as a statewide recreational trail, one of the few extant sections in San Diego County. Continuing along, you'll pass various side trails, nearly always associated with power line roads or other utility easements that run through the neighborhood. They offer access to Rice Canyon from the surrounding residential streets.

As you make your way down the canyon on a typical spring or early summer morning, you will be treated to an experience for all of your senses: The marine-layer clouds begin to part, and you'll breathe in salt-tinged air that pushes inland from south San Diego Bay. The California sagebrush plants coating the canyons exude a spicy fragrance fondly referred to as cowboy cologne—if brushed against, this attractive scent can linger even after you return home. The sounds of bird, cricket, and cicada songs waft on the breeze. White and yellow butterflies flit amid the wildflowers.

Go as far as you like on this easygoing trail. At 1.8 miles down from the start, you arrive at wide and busy H Street. Turn back at this point and enjoy a peaceful and quiet return with the same landscape in view, only from a different perspective.

TO THE TRAILHEAD
GPS Coordinates: N32° 38.685'   W117° 0.677'

Exit I-805 at H Street (Exit 7A) in Chula Vista. Drive 2.8 miles east to Paseo Ranchero and turn left (north). Go 0.2 mile north to Rancho Del Rey Parkway. Turn right (east) and drive 0.3 mile to the Rice Canyon Trailhead on the left, opposite Discovery Park.

49 Otay Lakes County Park

Trailhead Location: Eastern Chula Vista

Trail Use: Hiking, dog walking

Distance & Configuration: 0.9-mile out-and-back

Elevation Range: 520' at the start to 800'

Facilities: Water and restrooms at the start; tree-shaded lawn, pavilions, picnic tables, and playground

Highlights: Spectacular vista of Lower Otay Reservoir to the north, mountains to the east, and suburbs to the west

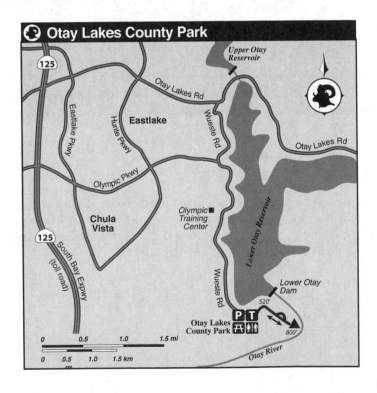

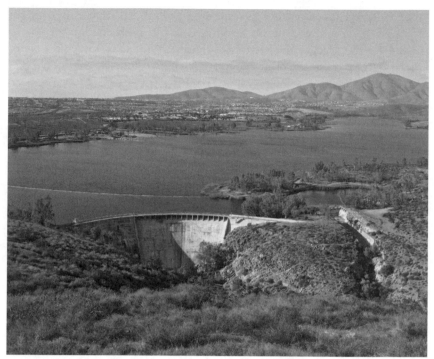

Lower Otay Lake and dam

DESCRIPTION

Otay Lakes County Park, on a hillside above the dam of Lower Otay Reservoir, was once a remote destination for most San Diegans. Now, due to the recent eastward spread of suburban development, the 78-acre park lies within only a few minutes' drive for tens of thousands of South Bay residents. Not only that, but renovation of the entire park has also turned it into a scenic spot for picnicking and special events with a fine view south into Mexico. Other amenities include horseshoe courts, multisensory trails, and a native plant garden. To see even farther, this hike engages you to make a short, steep climb to a hilltop. Day use is $3 per vehicle. Tickets are available at the entrance from a self-pay machine.

THE ROUTE

From the topmost parking lot inside Otay Lakes County Park, walk past a gate and go uphill on either an unpaved service road or on a parallel, zig-zagging foot trail. Either way, you soon arrive at a resting bench offering an expansive view. Continue on the eroded firebreak that runs straight up the slope. You'll end up on a rounded knoll, high enough for you to see the Pacific Ocean, the terrestrial ocean of rooftops covering eastern Chula Vista, and—when clear enough—the upper floors of downtown San Diego's skyscrapers.

For the most impressive vista, however, gaze north toward Lower Otay Reservoir, which spreads its waters far and wide, seemingly at your feet. To the east, the long ridge of Otay Mountain climbs steadily toward the 3,572-foot high point of that range. This upward pitch, however, is interrupted by the Otay River gorge immediately below you, so the rounded summit is as far as you can conveniently go.

You've traveled just short of 0.5 mile to reach and circle the top of this scenic knoll and gained a quick 300 feet of elevation too. When it's time to return, simply retrace your steps.

TO THE TRAILHEAD
GPS Coordinates: N32° 36.455'   W116° 55.747'

Exit the CA 125 toll road at Olympic Parkway (Exit 6) in east Chula Vista. Drive 2.7 miles east to Wueste Road and turn right (south). Continue south to the end of the road, where you'll find the entrance to Otay Lakes County Park.

Alternatively, exit I-805 at Orange Avenue (Exit 4) and head east on East Orange Avenue. In 0.6 mile, Orange becomes Olympic Parkway. Continue 6.2 miles and turn right (south) on Wueste Road, then drive 2.2 miles to the end of the road and the park entrance.

50 Imperial Beach

Trailhead Location: Imperial Beach

Trail Use: Hiking, dog walking

Distance & Configuration: 2-mile out-and-back

Elevation Range: Sea level throughout

Facilities: Nearest water and restrooms 1 mile north at Imperial Beach Pier

Highlights: A rare, undeveloped stretch of beach facing the Pacific Ocean; abundant birdlife

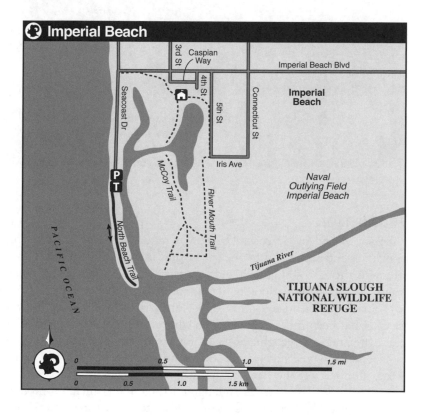

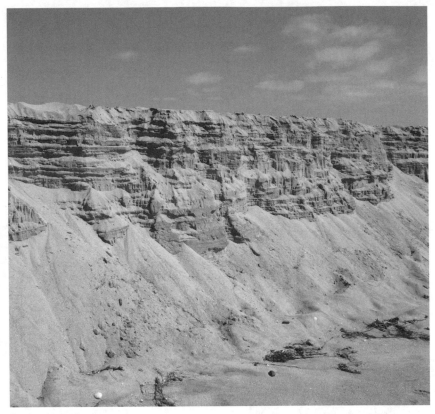

Sand castle walls

DESCRIPTION

At the south end of Seacoast Drive, a planked walkway and interpretive plaques introduce you to the green tidal marshlands of the Tijuana Estuary to the east. The marshlands are part of a 4-square-mile tideland expanse managed by various national, state, and local agencies. This is one of Southern California's most important coastal wetland areas simply because it has been mostly spared from commercial and housing developments. The area is a recognized haven for birds, and more than 400 species have been logged here so far. This is no surprise because the estuary is a key stopover on the Pacific Flyway—the equivalent of I-5 for bird-migration traffic. The marsh's endangered inhabitants include the light-footed Ridgway's rail and the California least tern. Visiting birds include ospreys, golden eagles, and peregrine falcons.

THE ROUTE

The walk itself begins with a little hop over rocks to the sandy beach. Modern houses and condominiums line the sandy strip to the north, but that's it for development as you travel south. Artificial dunes, off-limits to protect nesting terns, back up the beach to the left. At high tide, you could be edging close alongside those dunes, but low tide allows you to enjoy a wide, glassy-smooth expanse of wet sand, dimpled with rounded pebbles here and there.

At between 0.8 and 1 mile from the start, you reach the mouth of the Tijuana River. The distance may vary as the river outlet can shift where it comes through the barrier sand dunes. Pause to appreciate this river's work: One-quarter of its drainage area covers San Diego County, and three-quarters drains a substantial part of Baja California (including the city of Tijuana). When storm runoff courses down the river, it's fascinating to watch the outrushing turbid freshwater mixing with the incoming blue-green ocean waves. In winter, gulls and terns set up shop here, feeding in the water and wheeling overhead in great flocks. You may see an osprey

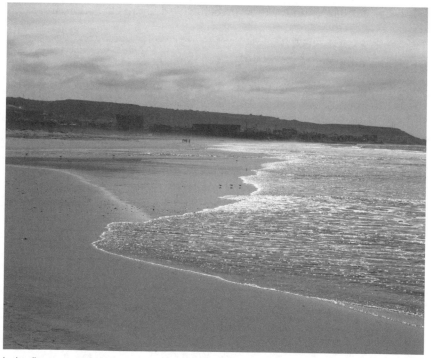

In the distance, you can see the Bullring by the Sea in Tijuana, Mexico.

plunge into the water to snatch up its next finny meal with its talons, lifting back up with a shake of its powerful wings to carry off a silvery mullet or other saltwater fish that may be nearly as heavy as itself.

Tijuana River water is of variable and often dubious quality, so it's not a great idea to wade or swim in or near the river's mouth. Most swimmers and surfers tend to hang out near the Imperial Beach Pier, where the beach is lifeguarded during the warmer months, and the water quality is better.

After some quality time river-gazing or shorebirding, return to your parked car the way you came.

If you have time after or before your walk, consider a visit to the Tijuana Estuary Visitor Center located at 301 Caspian Way between Third and Fourth Streets, one block south of Imperial Beach Boulevard. Jointly managed by the National Oceanic and Atmospheric Administration (NOAA), California State Parks, and U.S. Fish & Wildlife Service, the center is open Wednesday–Sunday, 10 a.m.–3 p.m. There is no entrance fee. Features include a diorama of the estuary, a large map showing migration on the Pacific Flyway, estuary trail maps, and bird identification pamphlets. If you would like to do a little birding while here, binoculars are available to borrow at no charge (unless they are being used for an education program).

TO THE TRAILHEAD

GPS Coordinates: N32° 33.994'   W117° 7.938'

Exit I-5 at Coronado Avenue (Exit 4) in south San Diego. Turn west toward the ocean. Coronado Avenue becomes Imperial Beach Boulevard in 1.1 miles as you enter the city of Imperial Beach. Continue another 1.65 miles to the end of Imperial Beach Boulevard, and turn left (south) at Seacoast Drive. Public parking spaces line both sides of Seacoast Drive, which dead-ends 0.7 mile south. Find a space as close to the end as possible to position yourself at the beginning of your walk. To get to the Tijuana Estuary Visitor Center, drive north on Seacoast back to Imperial, turn right (east) for two blocks, then turn right (south) on Third Street, then left on Caspian Way, and continue a half block to the entrance of the center's parking lot on your right.

INDEX

About the Authors

Jerry Schad
1949–2011
Jerry Schad's several careers encompassed interests ranging from astronomy and teaching to photography and writing. Schad held bachelor's and master's degrees in astronomy, taught physical science and astronomy at San Diego Mesa College, and chaired the Mesa College Physical Sciences Department.

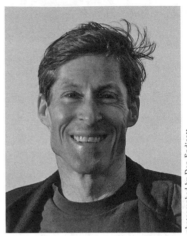

photographed by Don Endicott

Schad was the author of 16 books, including a college-level textbook for introductory physical science courses and the top-selling Afoot & Afield series of hiking guidebooks that cover nearly all of Southern California. He became interested in astronomy at age 12, took up astronomical photography a few years later, and had some 1,500 astronomical photographs published in media around the world.

Schad's outdoor column, "Roam-O-Rama," was published weekly in the *San Diego Reader* 1993–2011, and his *San Diego Reader* blog, "Outdoor San Diego," kept San Diegans up-to-date on a variety of natural events in the sky and on Earth.

At one time, Schad ran a 100-mile trail race across the Sierra Nevada in 24 hours. He also bicycled 352 miles from San Jose to the outskirts of Los Angeles in even less time.

In the last year of his life, Schad enjoyed spending time with his wife, Peg Reiter, as they walked, hiked, traveled, and enjoyed time in their high-rise residential tower in downtown San Diego.

In the months preceding his death at age 61 from kidney cancer, Schad worked tirelessly and with courageous joy and spirit to complete the final stages of the first edition of this book.

Don Endicott

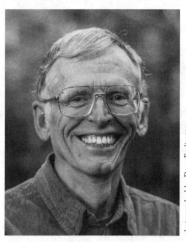

photographed by Dave Endicott

A retired civilian research engineer in the field of Navy communications and network technologies, Don Endicott discovered a second career as a volunteer naturalist. He is an NAI Certified Interpretive Guide, presenting multimedia campground and visitor center talks at Anza-Borrego Desert State Park, Cuyamaca Rancho State Park, Mission Trails Regional Park, and San Diego County Parks. Endicott is a regular volunteer field contributor at Cabrillo National Monument for faunal surveys and intertidal interpretation and monitors a wild breeding pair of peregrine falcons at Cabrillo National Monument. An avid hiker and climber, he has enjoyed more than 50 years exploring and photographing wildlife and remote wilderness settings throughout California and the western states and has stood atop many of the region's highest summits. Prior to retirement, Endicott served as a Sierra Club National Outings Leader.

A long-time hiking and running companion of Jerry Schad's, Endicott partnered on field research leading to the first edition of *Afoot & Afield: San Diego County*. He advised and supported fieldwork for the fifth edition of the book with coauthor Scott Turner. Endicott contributed hike write-ups and photography for "Roam-O-Rama" and the recently published San Diego Natural History Museum's *Coast to Cactus: The Canyoneer Trail Guide to San Diego Outdoors*. His photography has been featured in print and online publications for Anza-Borrego Desert State Park, Cabrillo National Monument, Yosemite National Park, and the Yosemite Conservancy. This is his first book.

Other Books by Jerry Schad from Wilderness Press

Afoot & Afield Orange County

In 87 hikes in the parks, preserves, designated open spaces, and public lands surrounding Orange County's densely populated coastal plain, this up-to-date fourth edition provides fresh inspiration for trips along the coast from Huntington Beach to San Clemente, in the rugged Santa Ana Mountains, and through the foothills from Anaheim to the Santa Rosa Plateau Ecological Reserve.
ISBN 978-0-89997-757-7

Afoot & Afield Los Angeles County

This guide covers all the best LA adventures, from strolling along Point Dume to trekking up a mountain on Santa Catalina Island. Choose from 200 trips to explore the City of Angels' own backyard, traveling through a variety of climate zones and revealing a remarkably diverse array of plant and animal life.
ISBN 978-0-89997-499-6

Afoot & Afield San Diego County

Updated by Scott Turner, the fifth edition of San Diego County's classic hiking guidebook features 282 trips, ranging from short, self-guiding nature trails to challenging peak climbs and canyon treks. The book encompasses almost all public—and a few private—lands within San Diego County, including Anza-Borrego Desert State Park, Cleveland National Forest, the Cuyamaca Mountains, and numerous county and city parks.
ISBN 978-0-89997-801-7

101 Hikes in Southern California

Updated by David Harris, the third edition of this book proves that there's more to SoCal than theme parks and strip malls. This guide offers an incredible selection of exciting trips, from the San Gabriel Mountains to the Anza-Borrego Desert and everywhere in between, covering scores of hidden places just beyond the urban horizon.
ISBN 978-0-89997-716-4

For ordering information, contact your local
bookseller or Wilderness Press.
wildernesspress.com